Color Atlas of Acupuncture
Body Points, Ear Points, Trigger Points

Hans-Ulrich Hecker, M.D.
Physician in Private Practice
Kiel, Germany

Angelika Steveling, M.D.
Physician in Private Practice
Essen, Germany

Elmar Peuker, M.D.
Institute of Microtherapy
University of Witten-Herdecke
Bochum, Germany

Jörg Kastner, M.D.
Academy for Acupuncture
and TCM, Bochum, Germany

Kay Liebchen, M.D.
Physician in Private Practice
Fleckeby, Germany

With the collaboration of
Stefan Kopp, Gustav Peters, Michael Hammes

Thieme
Stuttgart · New York

Library of Congress Cataloging-in-Publication Data is available from the publisher.

Graphics by Martin Wunderlich, Kiel
Anatomical drawings by
Rüdiger Bremert, München
Photographs by Axel Nickolaus, Kiel

Translated by Ursula Vielkind, Ph.D.,
Dundas, Canada

This book is an authorized translation of the German edition published and copyrighted 1999 by Hippokrates Verlag, Stuttgart, Germany.
Title of the German edition: Taschenlehrbuch der Akupunktur: Körperpunkte, Ohrpunkte, Triggerpunkte.

© 2001 Georg Thieme Verlag,
Rüdigerstraße 14,
D-70469 Stuttgart, Germany
Thieme New York, 333 Seventh Avenue,
New York, NY 10001, USA

Cover design: Martina Berge,
Erbach-Ernsbach

Typesetting by primustype Robert Hurler GmbH, D-73274 Notzingen
Printed in Germany by
Staudigl, Donauwörth

ISBN 3-13-125221-9 (GTV)
ISBN 0-86577-938-4 (TNY)   3   4   5

Preface

For the first time, there is now a pocket atlas covering the major body and ear acupuncture points as well as the most frequently occurring trigger points. With this book we comply with the requests of many physicians to provide reference material that makes possible quick orientation during daily practice. The authors come from diverse fields of specialization, thus ensuring the highest competence possible.

The book consistently follows the visual-didactic presentation concept (VISDAK, visuell-didaktisches Aufarbeitungskonzept). This concept has already gained recognition through the two textbooks, *Acupuncture of Ear, Skull, Mouth, and Hand* and *The Acupuncture Points*. This type of presentation has been borne out of a large number of positive responses and serves as a useful building block when learning new and complex material. The description of the locations of acupuncture points follows the style of the localization specifications effective in China as they have been described in the usual standard publications for foreigners. The details are presented using the latest anatomical nomenclature. In particular, practical advice for quick orientation during localization is emphasized. The action of individual points is described according to both the conventional medical indications and the traditional Chinese avenues of action.

The basics presented here will help the targeted preparation for an exam and will also serve the actively practicing physician as a quick reference for orientation. The experienced acupuncturist will find interesting details for precise point localization as far as anatomical guiding structures are concerned. The major trigger points are described in connection with acupuncture points according to practical relevance. Gnathological aspects are particularly emphasized as they play a major role within the holistic approach.

The selection of acupuncture points is based on the experience of the physicians participating in this book project, all of whom have been using acupuncture in their practice for many years and/or are participating in university level education in acupuncture. We would like to thank all those who have been involved in the realization of this book: Mr. Rüdiger Bremert for his excellent anatomical drawings, Mr. Axel Nickolaus for the photographic illustrations and Mr. Martin Wunderlich for the professional graphic design. Our special thanks are due to Ms Helga Gilleberg for all the typing–from the first draft to the original version prior to printing. Our thanks go to Thieme International Editorial and Production Departments, especially for the opportunity of using four-color printing and for the customer-friendly price-performance ratio.

Kiel, Münster, Bochum, Damp, and Essen, April 2001

Hans-Ulrich Hecker
Angelika Steveling
Elmar Peuker
Jörg Kastner
Kay Liebchen

The Authors

Hecker, Hans-Ulrich, M.D.
Medical specialist in general medicine, naturopathy, homeopathy.
Lecturer in Naturopathy and Acupuncture, Christian Albrecht University, Kiel, Germany.
Research Director of Education in Naturopathy and Acupuncture, Academy of Continuing Medical Education of the Regional Medical Association of Schleswig-Holstein.
Certified Medical Quality Manager.
Assessor of the European Foundation of Quality Management (EFQM)

Steveling, Angelika, M.D.
Chiropractor, NLP Practitioner, Essen, Germany.
Lecturer of the German Society of Physicians for Acupuncture (DÄGfA).

Peuker, Elmar, M.D.
Consultant of anatomy.
Head of the Department of Traditional Medicine at the Institute of Microtherapy, University of Witten-Herdecke, Germany.
Head of the Complementary Medicine Study Group, Department of Anatomy, University of Münster, Germany.

Kastner, Jörg, M.P.
Education in internal medicine, Sports medicine, naturopathy.
Founder and Head of the Academy for Acupuncture and TCM, Bochum, Germany.
Research Director of Education in Acupuncture and TCM, Academy for Continuing Medical Education of the Regional Medical Association of Westphalia-Lippe.
Lecturer of the Complementary Medicine Study Group, Department of Anatomy, Wilhelm University of Westphalia, Münster, Germany.

Liebchen, Kay, M.D.
Medical specialist in orthopedics, chiropractic, physiotherapy, special pain management, sports medicine.
Instructor and lecturer for continuing education in special pain management, Damp, Germany.
Expert representative on the examining board for special pain management, Damp, Germany.
Guest lecturer of the German Society of Physicians for Acupuncture (DÄGfA).

Collaborators

Kopp, Stefan, D. M.D.
Oral surgeon, orthodontist.
Senior Physician of the Orthopedic Outpatient Clinic, Friedrich Schiller University, Jena, Germany.
Head of the Temporomandibular Joint Consulting Practice.
Head of the Interdisciplinary Pain Management Consulting Practice.

Peters, Gustav, M.D.
Medical specialist in general medicine, homeopathy, and chiropractic, Hankensbüttel, Germany.
Lecturer of the German Society of Physicians for Acupuncture (DÄGfA).
Focus on ear acupuncture/auriculomedicine.

Hammes, Michael, Physician
Residence physician, Neurological Clinic of the Technical University of Munich, Munich, Germany.
Lecturer of the German Society of Physicians for Acupuncture (DÄGfA).

Contents

■ Part 1:
Body Acupuncture Points

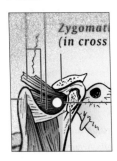

■ Part 2:
Ear Acupuncture Points

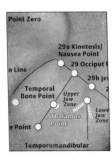

■ Part 2:
Ear Acupuncture Points

■ Part 3:
Trigger Points

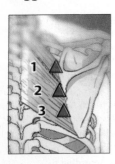

■ **Part 3:**
Trigger Points

■ **Part 3:**
Trigger Points

List of Points

Localization of Acupuncture Points

In China, acupuncture points are primarily localized using proportional measurements expressed in **body Cun**. The unit of measurement, Cun, is further divided into Fen so that 1 Cun equals 10 Fen.

For various body regions, proportional measurements are given in Cun. For example, the distance between elbow crease and wrist measures 12 Cun. In the lower arm region, specifications in Cun are always made according to these proportional measurements given as a total number of Cun. For example, a distance of 4 Cun from the dorsal wrist crease means that the point lies proximal to the wrist crease at one-third of the total distance between elbow crease and wrist.

The proportional orientation takes into account individual variations in body proportions. This is of particular importance in the abdominal region. For example, 1 Cun cranial to the symphysis does not mean that the point (CV 3) is found one width of a patient's thumb above the symphysis. Instead, the total distance between the navel and upper margin of the symphysis has to be subdivided into five equal sections (e.g., by using a graded rubber band as a measuring tape). The point to be localized lies proximal to one-fifth of the total distance between the navel and upper margin of the symphysis. Only if orientation according to the proportional measurements in **body Cun** is not feasible, is the patient's **thumb Cun** used as a unit of measurement.

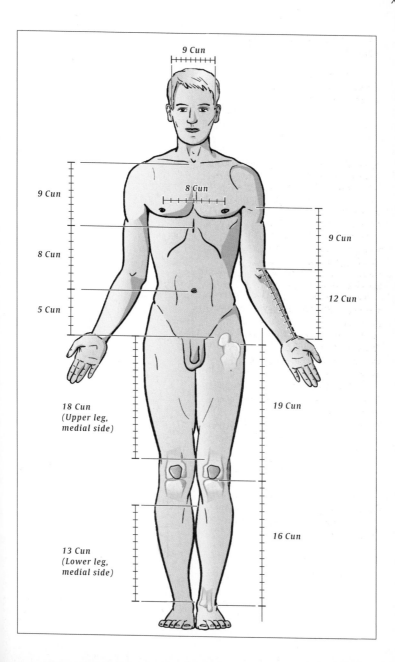

9 Cun

8 Cun

9 Cun

8 Cun

5 Cun

9 Cun

12 Cun

18 Cun
(Upper leg, medial side)

19 Cun

13 Cun
(Lower leg, medial side)

16 Cun

The Proportional Measurement Based on Body Cun

Face
The distance between both acupoints St 8 measures 9 Cun.

Thorax
The distance between the sternal manubrium and base of the xiphoid process measures 9 Cun. However, orientation in the thoracic region is based on intercostal spaces (ICS). The transition between sternal manubrium and sternal body is clearly palpable in the area of the sternal synchondrosis. The 2nd rib lies lateral to this transition. The 2nd ICS lies caudal to the 2nd rib.

The distance between the two mamillae measures 8 Cun.

Abdomen
The distance between the base of the xiphoid process and the navel measures 8 Cun.

The distance between the navel and the upper margin of the symphysis measures 5 Cun.

Upper Extremity
The distance between the elbow crease and the upper fold of the armpit measures 9 Cun.

The distance between the elbow crease and the palmar wrist crease measures 12 Cun.

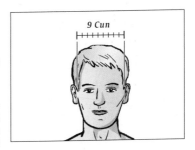

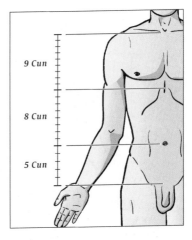

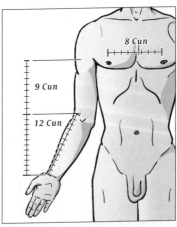

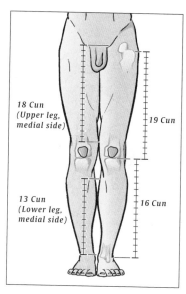

18 Cun
(Upper leg,
medial side)

19 Cun

13 Cun
(Lower leg,
medial side)

16 Cun

Lower Extremity

Lateral side: The distance between the highest point of the greater trochanter and the knee-joint crevice (lower edge of patella) measures 19 Cun.

The distance between the knee-joint crevice and the highest point of the lateral malleolus measures 16 Cun.

Medial side: The distance between the upper margin of the symphysis and the transition of the femoral shaft to the medial epicondyle measures 18 Cun.

The distance between the transition of the tibial shaft to the medial condyle of tibia and the medial malleolus measures 13 Cun.

Dorsal Body

The distance between both mastoid processes measures 9 Cun.

The distance between the dorsal midline through the spinous processes and medial margin of the scapula at the attachment of the scapular spine measures 3 Cun (in a patient with the arms hanging down).

Lateral Head

The distance between the middle of the frontal hairline and the middle of the dorsal hairline measures 12 Cun.

The distance between the middle of the eyebrow and the frontal hairline measures 3 Cun.

The distance between the spinous process of C7 and the dorsal hairline measures 3 Cun.

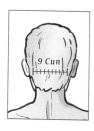

9 Cun

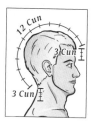

12 Cun

3 Cun

3 Cun

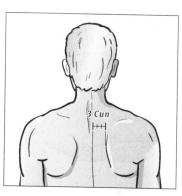

3 Cun

The Proportional Measurement Based on Finger Cun

The distance between the palmar crease of the proximal interphalangeal joint and the palmar crease of the distal interphalangeal joint of the middle finger measures 1 Cun.

At its greatest width, the thumb measures 1 Cun.

Middle and index fingers together measure 1.5 Cun in the most distal region.

Middle, index, and ring fingers together measure 2 Cun in the most distal region.

Middle, index, ring, and little fingers together measure 3 Cun in the widest area over the knuckles.

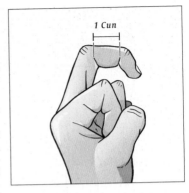

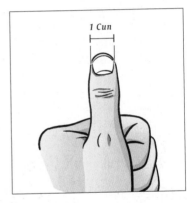

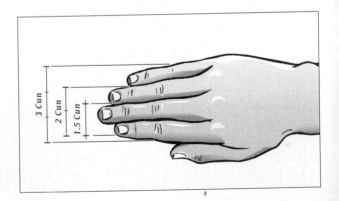

Part 1: Body Acupuncture Points

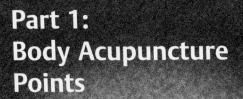

Coronoid process

Lateral pterygoid muscle

Mandibular notch

Zygomatic arch (in cross section)

St 7

Condylar process (in cross section)

Major Points of the Lung Meridian

Lu 1: Front Collecting Point (Mu Point) of the Lung.

Lu 5: Sedation point.

Lu 7: Connecting Point (Luo Point). Opening Point of the Conception Vessel Ren Mai.

Lu 9: Source Point (Yuan Point). Tonification point. Master Point of the blood vessels.

Lu 11: Local point.

Points Associated with the Lung Meridian

Lu 1: Front Collecting Point (Mu Point) of the Lung.

B 13: Back Transporting Point (Back Shu Point) of the Lung.

Coupling Relationships of the Lung Meridian

Top-to-bottom coupling:
Lung–Spleen

Yin-Yang coupling:
Lung–Large Intestine

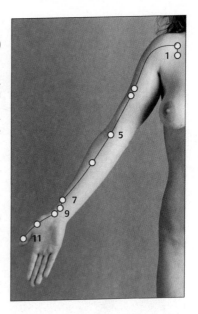

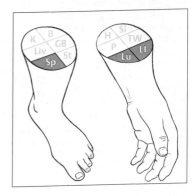

Lu 1 "Zhong Fu"
"Central Residence"
("Central Mansion")
Front Collecting Point (Mu Point)
of the Lung

Location: 6 Cun lateral to the median line, 1 Cun below the clavicle, slightly medial to the caudal border of the coracoid process, at the level of the first intercostal space (ICS 1).

!

● To find the coracoid process, palpate in cranial direction along the anterior fold of the armpit until you feel a distinct bony marker. The coracoid process is best palpated when gliding the finger at the caudal margin of the clavicle in lateral direction. In front of the bony structure to be searched for, the finger slides into a soft depression (absence of the bony ribs). The coracoid process is located slightly further laterally.

Differentiation between the coracoid process and lesser tubercle of humerus: When the arm is rotated slightly outward and the elbow flexed, the coracoid process does not move, while the lesser tubercle of humerus immediately follows the movement.

Advice: Lu 1 lies in the area of tendon insertions of the smaller pectoral muscle, biceps muscle of arm (short head) and coracobrachial muscle; these muscles are often shortened and sensitive to pressure in cases of poor posture in the thoracic region.

Depth of needling: 0.3 to 0.5 Cun, obliquely in lateral direction.

This point belongs to the dangerous acupuncture points because of the risk of causing a pneumothorax (especially if there is an emphysema vesicle in older patients) by improper needling in mediodorsal direction. The point should only be needled in laterodorsal direction, i.e., in the direction of the coracoid process, or tangentially along the coracoid process.

Indication: Diseases of the respiratory tract, cough and bronchitis with phlegm, bronchial asthma, tonsillitis, shoulder–arm syndrome, pain in the chest.

Action in Traditional Chinese Medicine (TCM): Used predominantly in the acute phase of symptom patterns of Congestion or Stagnation; regulates the circulation of Lung Qi and stimulates its descending, expels Heat and Phlegm Heat from the Lung, invigorates Lung Qi, clears and opens the Upper Warmer.

Lu 1 + Lu 5: Sedative effect; expel Lung Heat and Phlegm Heat.

Lu 1 + Lu 7: In cases of pain, stiffness in the chest, neck, and shoulder girdle.

Lu 1 + Lu 7 + CV 17: Unresolved grief, depression, melancholia.

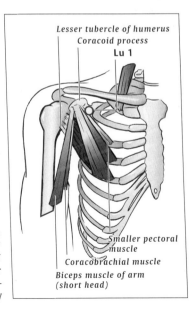

Lesser tubercle of humerus
Coracoid process
Lu 1

Smaller pectoral muscle
Coracobrachial muscle
Biceps muscle of arm (short head)

○ **Lu 5 "Chi Ze"**
   "Foot Marsh"
   Sedation Point

Location: Radial to the biceps tendons in the elbow crease.

> **!** The biceps tendons are best found when the lower arm is flexed and supine.

Depth of needling: 0.5 to 1 Cun, perpendicularly.

Indication: Bronchial asthma, bronchitis, croup, tonsillitis, epicondylopathy, skin diseases; possibly microphlebotomy in case of Congestion diseases, possibly moxibustion in case of weakness (caution: asthma, ragweed allergy); pain and swelling on the inside of the knee, pain in the shoulder.
H. Schmidt: Repeated moxa in case of croup.
J. Bischko: Facial skin diseases.

Action in TCM: Used predominantly in symptom patterns of Congestion; cools Heat in the Upper Warmer, clears Lung Heat, expels Lung Phlegm, regulates Lung Qi and stimulates its descending, relaxes the tendons.
Lu 5 + St 40: Sedative effect; acute and chronic bronchitis with lots of phlegm.
Lu 5 + K 6: Tonification effect; Yin Deficiency of Lung, e.g., chronic dryness of the throat.

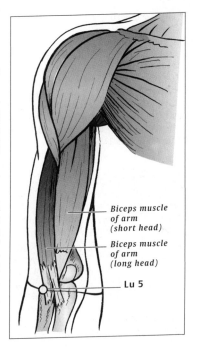

Biceps muscle of arm (short head)

Biceps muscle of arm (long head)

Lu 5

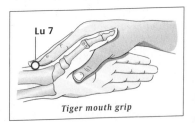

Lu 7

Tiger mouth grip

○ **Lu 7 "Lie Que"**
"Broken Sequence"
("Branching Crevice")
Connecting Point (Luo Point)
Opening Point of the Conception
Vessel, Ren Mai

Location: Radiolateral on the lower arm, in a V-shaped groove proximal to the styloid process of radius, 1.5 Cun proximal to the crease of the wrist.

!

● This groove is created by the tendon of the brachioradial muscle which inserts here at the radius under the long abductor muscle of thumb.

The tiger mouth grip may be used here for finding this point (see fig. at bottom of p. 4). Lu 7 lies on the border between the inside and outside of the lower arm, right in front of the tip of the examiner's index finger.
As a point of a Yin Meridian, Point Lu 7 still lies just within the Yin region.

!

● To find the point, avoid forming an angle between hand and lower arm regions of both arms when using the tiger mouth grip.

Method of needling: Lift the skin by forming a skin fold proximal to the styloid process of radius, then insert the needle in the lifted fold in oblique proximal direction.

Depth of needling: 0.5 to 1 Cun, obliquely in proximal direction.

Indication: Bronchial asthma, bronchitis, cough, arthralgia of the wrist, migraine, cephalalgia, autonomic dysregulation, tics in the facial area, stuffy nose, facial paralysis.

Action in TCM: Stimulates the dispersing and descending of Lung Qi; expels pathogenic factors, particularly exterior Wind and Wind Cold, and to a lesser extent also Wind Heat; stimulates sweating, opens the nose, communicates with the Large Intestine. The point is used in cases of mental and emotional problems resulting from Lung Disharmony, e.g., unresolved grief, repressed emotions, depression.
Lu 7 + LI 20: Stuffy or running nose, cough.

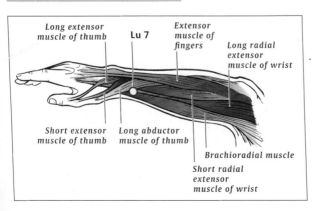

Long extensor muscle of thumb   Lu 7   Extensor muscle of fingers   Long radial extensor muscle of wrist

Short extensor muscle of thumb   Long abductor muscle of thumb

Brachioradial muscle
Short radial extensor muscle of wrist

○ **Lu 9 "Tai Yuan"**
"Greater Abyss" ("Great Gulf")
Source Point (Yuan Point)
Tonification Point
Master Point of the Blood Vessels

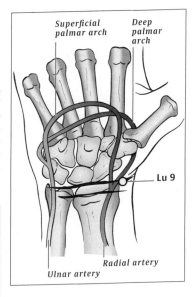

Superficial palmar arch

Deep palmar arch

Lu 9

Radial artery

Ulnar artery

Location: Radial side of the flexion crease of the wrist, lateral to the radial artery. Of the existing wrist creases, one should use the one lying between radius and ulna on one side and the bones of the wrist on the other side. The wrist crease lying distal to the clearly palpable end of the styloid process of radius should be selected.

! The desired position of the needle is close to the radial artery. This results in a direct effect on the perivascular sympathetic neurovascular plexus. (Explanation of the effect of acupuncture according to König and Wancura: Lu 9 is the Master Point for blood vessels.) The position of the needle is therefore correct when the needle pulses. From now on, however, there must be no more stimulation with the needle, i.e., the sedation method should not be used. As long as bypass circulation through the ulnar artery exists (to be established by prior palpation of the ulnar artery), accidental puncture of the radial artery has no effect whatsoever if subsequently compressed.

Depth of needling: 2 to 3 mm, perpendicularly.

Indication: Diseases of the respiratory tract, bronchial asthma, chronic bronchitis, cough, circulatory disorders, peripheral arterial occlusive disease, Raynaud's disease, affections of the wrist.

Action in TCM: The most important point for tonifying Lung Qi and Lung Yin; promotes and regulates the circulation of Lung Qi, alleviates cough, removes Phlegm, clears Heat from Lung and Liver, expels Wind, promotes circulation of Blood.

Lu 9 + B 13 + St 36: Very effective in chronic Lung Qi Deficiency.

Lu 9 + CV 6: Generalized Qi Deficiency, such as chronic fatigue.

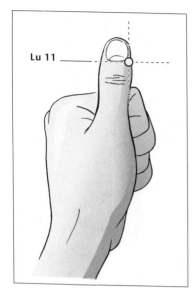

Lu 11

Lu 11 "Shao Shang"
"Lesser Metal" ("Young Shang")

Location: Radial angle of the thumbnail (Chinese), ulnar angle of the thumbnail (*J. Bischko*). As shown in the figure, the thumbnail point is localized on the intersection of the vertical and horizontal lines of the nail.

Depth of needling: 1 to 2 mm, perpendicularly; let bleed if necessary.

Indication: Inflammatory diseases of the throat.
J. Bischko: Master Point for diseases of the throat (see remark), possibly with microphlebotomy in case of acute symptoms.
Remark: Apart from the eight proper Master Points (Liv 13, CV 12 and 17, B 11 and 17, GB 34 and 39, Lu 9), *J. Bischko* described about 40 additional "Master Points."

Action in TCM: Cools Lung Heat, expels exterior and interior Wind, eliminates Wind Heat, benefits the throat, frees the senses, awakens from unconsciousness, regulates descending Lung Qi.

Major Points of the Large Intestine Meridian

LI 1: Local point.
LI 4: Source Point (Yuan Point).
LI 10: Local point.
LI 11: Tonification point.
LI 14: Local point.
LI 15: Local point.
LI 20: Local point.

Points Associated with the Large Intestine Meridian

St 25: Front Collecting Point (Mu Point) of the Large Intestine.
B 25: Back Transporting Point (Back Shu Point) of the Large Intestine.
St 37: Lower Sea Point (Lower He Point) of the Large Intestine.

Coupling Relationships of the Large Intestine Meridian

Top-to-bottom coupling:
Large Intestine–Stomach

Yang-Yin coupling:
Large Intestine–Lung

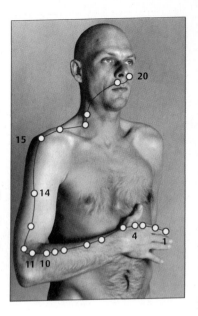

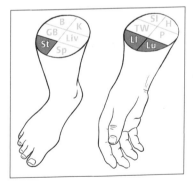

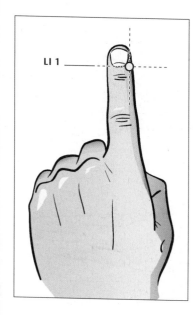

● **LI 1 "Shang Yang"**
   "Metal Yang"

Location: Radial corner of the nail of the index finger (for exact localization of starting and end points of the meridians of the hand, see Point Lu 11).

Depth of needling: 1 to 2 mm, perpendicularly, let bleed if necessary.

Indication: Acute fever, acute toothache, acute inflammation of the throat; important analgetic point.
J. Bischko: Master Point for toothache.
Remark: For more details on Master Points according to *J. Bischko*, see Point Lu 11.

Action in TCM: Expels exterior pathogenic factors, such as Heat, Wind Heat, Wind Cold; benefits the throat, clears the Mind and the eyes.

● **LI 4 "He Gu"**

**"Joining Valley" ("Connected Valleys," "Enclosed Valley")
Source Point (Yuan Point)**

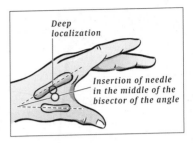

Deep localization

Insertion of needle in the middle of the bisector of the angle

Location: There are several possibilities for localizing this most commonly used acupuncture point:

1. When the thumb is abducted, the point lies halfway on the line connecting the middle of metacarpal bone I with the middle of metacarpal bone II. The needle is pushed forward about 0.5 to 1 Cun in the direction of the lower surface of the shaft of metacarpal bone II.
2. When the thumb is adducted, the highest point of the dorsal interosseous muscle I, which is contracted during adduction and pushed upward by the adductor muscle of thumb, is used for needling. After inserting the needle, the hand is immediately allowed to relax and the needle is pushed forward approximately 0.5 to 1 Cun toward the middle of the lower surface of metacarpal bone II. This kind of localization can only be used when the highest point of the muscle bulge lies in the middle of metacarpal bone II.
3. When the thumb is abducted, palpation is carried out in the direction of metacarpal bone II with the other hand's angled phalange of thumb. This localization aid serves particularly to feel the De Qi sensation. The angled thumb is pressed moderately firmly against the lower surface of metacarpal bone II. Point LI 4 in the lower figure thus corresponds to the deep localization of the point.

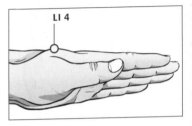

LI 4

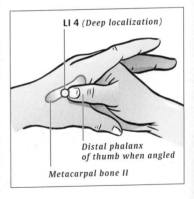

LI 4 *(Deep localization)*

Distal phalanx of thumb when angled

Metacarpal bone II

Depth of needling: 0.5 to 1 Cun, slightly oblique in proximal direction toward the palm.

Indication: This is the most important analgetic Point which affects the entire body; fever, beginning of feverish colds, hemiplegia, acne, eczema, affections of the head region (pain, inflammation, allergic reactions), facial paralysis, abdominal symptoms, general effect on metabolism, labor-promoting effect, dysmenorrhea.

! Point LI 4 must not be needled during pregnancy, except to facilitate birth.

Action in TCM: Expels exterior pathogenic factors, especially Wind; relieves the Exterior of the body, purges Cold, expels Heat and Summer Heat, alleviates pain, calms the Mind (Shen), regulates Qi of Large Intestine, harmonizes ascending and descending Qi, disperses Lung Qi.

○ **LI 10 "Shou San Li"**
"Arm Three Miles" ("Hand Three Li")

Location: 2 Cun distal to Point LI 11 on the line connecting Points LI 5 and LI 11 in the long radial extensor muscle of wrist (with deep needling into the supinator muscle).

! The point is searched for with the lower arm slightly flexed and the thumb pointing upward.

Depth of needling: 1 to 2 Cun, perpendicularly.

Indication: General tonification point (moxa); lateral humeral epicondylitis (tennis elbow), paresis of the upper extremity.
H. Schmidt: Inflammatory facial rash, nasal furuncle (moxa).
J. Bischko: Test point for obstipation.

Action in TCM: Removes obstructions from the Large Intestine Meridian, resolves stagnation of Stomach and Intestine.

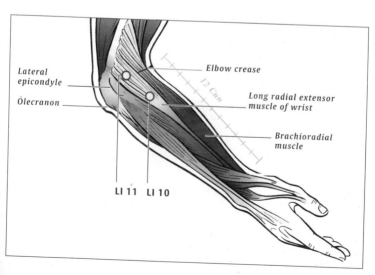

Lateral epicondyle

Ólecranon

Elbow crease

12 Cun

Long radial extensor muscle of wrist

Brachioradial muscle

LI 11   LI 10

○ LI 11 "Qu Chi"
"Crooked Pond" ("Bent Pond")
Tonification Point

Location: Lateral to the radial end of the elbow flexion crease when the lower arm is flexed at a right angle, in a depression between the end of the elbow crease and the lateral epicondyle in the region of the long radial extensor muscle. The point lies between Point Lu 5 and the lateral epicondyle of humerus.

> ! If there are two creases, a light pull at the skin toward the olecranon will identify the crease to be used.

Depth of needling: 1 to 2 Cun, perpendicularly.

Indication: Lateral humeral epicondylitis, paresis of the upper extremity, general immunomodulating effect, homeostatic effect, reducing fever; skin disorders, allergic disorders, abdominal disorders, soft or liquid stools with bad odor (traveler's diarrhea). Microphlebotomy in cases of pharyngitis and laryngitis.

Action in TCM: Expels Wind, clears Wind Heat, clears Heat, relieves the Exterior of the body, regulates Large Intestine, cools Blood, removes Dampness; regulates Qi, Blood, and Lung Qi; calms Liver Yang and Liver Fire; benefits the tendons, muscles, and joints.

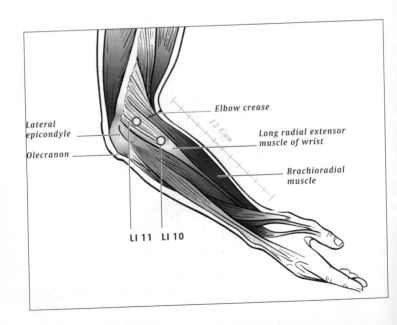

Elbow crease

Lateral epicondyle

Olecranon

12 Cun

Long radial extensor muscle of wrist

Brachioradial muscle

LI 11   LI 10

○ **LI 14 "Bi Nao"**
   "Arm and Scapula"
   ("Middle of Upper Arm")

Location: At the insertion of the medial part of the deltoid muscle. The point lies on the line connecting Points LI 11 and LI 15, 2 Cun caudal to the anterior end of the armpit fold. The insertion of the deltoid muscle can be easily localized when the arm is abducted.

Depth of needling: 0.5 to 1.5 Cun, perpendicularly.

Indication: Periarthritis of shoulder, neuralgia and paresis of the upper extremity.

Action in TCM: Removes obstructions from the Large Intestine Meridian.
LI 14, 15, 16 + LI 4 + St 38: Shoulder–arm syndrome along the Large Intestine Meridian.

○ **LI 15 "Jian Yu"**
   "Shoulder Transporting Point"
   ("Shoulder Blade")

Location: When the arm is abducted, two depressions are created slightly ventral and dorsal to the acromion. Point LI 15 lies in the region of the ventral depression immediately below the ventral pole of the acromion.
Remark: The two depressions ventral and dorsal to the acromion have the following anatomical explanation:
The deltoid muscle consists of three parts:

the clavicular part,
the acromial part,
and the spinal part (belonging to the spine of scapula).

At each location where two parts originate, a depression forms below the acromion at the end of the clearly visible muscle groove.

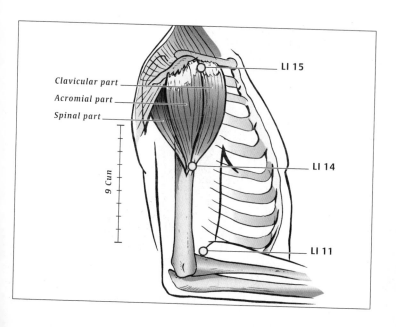

Clavicular part
Acromial part
Spinal part

LI 15

LI 14

LI 11

9 Cun

! The ventral pole of the acromion is best found by palpating along the ventral clavicular region in lateral direction. The dorsal pole of the acromion becomes palpable when the scapular spine is followed in lateral direction.

Depth of needling: 0.5 Cun, perpendicularly, or 1 to 2 Cun in oblique distal direction.

● There is a risk of piercing the shoulder joint when needling in vertical direction.

Indication: Periarthritis of shoulder (frozen shoulder), paresis of upper extremity, neuralgia in the upper extremity. *J. Bischko:* Master Point for paresis of upper extremity (for more details on Master Points according to *J. Bischko*, see Point Lu 11).

H. Schmidt: In case of hemiplegia, daily moxa from day 7 after paralysis; prophylactic effect against muscle atrophy.

Action in TCM: Expels Wind from all four extremities, promotes the flow of Qi in the meridian and collateral vessels, benefits tendons and joints.

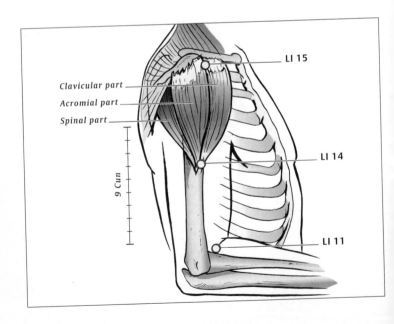

Clavicular part
Acromial part
Spinal part

9 Cun

LI 15

LI 14

LI 11

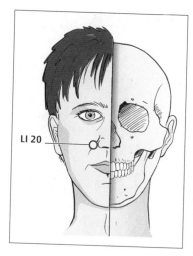

LI 20

○ **LI 20 "Ying Xiang"**
"Welcome Fragrance"
("Welcoming Perfume")

Location: Approximately 5 Fen lateral to the middle of the nasal wing, in the nasolabial groove.

Depth of needling: 3 to 8 mm, obliquely in craniomedial direction.
Advice: Cleanliness is particularly important in this region. Under no circumstances should needling be undertaken in infected regions. Point LI 20 lies close to the angular vein which drains the blood from the facial area above the lips. The angular vein possesses anastomoses to the ophthalmic vein and therefore has connections to the cavernous sinus. In case of infection, there is a risk of sinus thrombosis and central inflammatory processes.

Indication: Rhinitis, sinusitis, anosmia, toothache, facial paralysis, trigeminal neuralgia.

Action in TCM: Expels exterior Wind, relieves the nose, cools Wind Heat in the Yang Ming axis.

Major Points of the Stomach Meridian

St 2: Local point.
St 6: Local point.
St 7: Local point.
St 8: Local point.
St 25: Front Collecting Point (Mu Point) of the Large Intestine.
St 34: Cleft Point (Xi Point).
St 35: Local point.
St 36: Lower Sea Point (Lower He Point) of the Stomach.
St 38: Local point with remote effect on the shoulder.
St 40: Connecting Point (Luo Point).
St 41: Tonification point.
St 44: Peripheral pain point.

Points Associated with the Stomach Meridian

CV 12: Front Collecting Point (Mu Point) of the Stomach.
B 21: Back Transporting Point (Back Shu Point) of the Stomach.
St 36: Lower Sea Point (Lower He Point) of the Stomach.

Coupling Relationships of the Stomach Meridian

Top-to-bottom coupling:
Large Intestine–Stomach

Yang-Yin coupling:
Stomach–Spleen

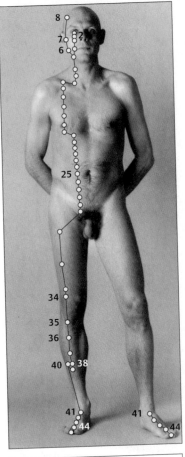

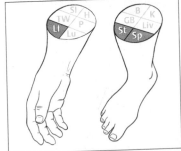

○ **St 2 "Si Bai"**
   "Four Whites"

Location: Above the infraorbital foramen below the pupilla when looking straight ahead.

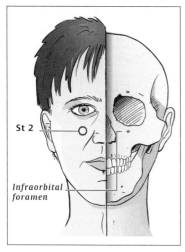

St 2

Infraorbital foramen

! ● The infraorbital foramen usually lies slightly medial to the vertical line drawn through the middle of the pupilla when looking straight ahead, approximately in the middle of the total length of the nose.

Depth of needling: 0.3 to 0.5 Cun, perpendicularly.
Advice: Regarding the risks resulting from needling in infected regions within the drainage area of the angular vein, see Point LI 20.

Indication: Eye diseases, migraine, rhinitis, sinusitis, facial paralysis, trigeminal neuralgia.

Action in TCM: Dispels exterior Wind, relieves the nose, cools Wind Heat in the Yang Ming axis.

○ **St 6 "Jia Che"**
   "Jaw Chariot" ("Mandibular Angle")

Location: 1 Cun cranial and ventral to the angle of the lower jaw. The masseter muscle can be palpated here when biting.

! ● The localization of Point St 6 corresponds to that of a common trigger point in the insertion of the masseter muscle.

Depth of needling: 0.3 Cun, perpendicularly.

Indication: Myofacial pain dysfunction (Costen's syndrome), facial pain, facial paralysis, trigeminal neuralgia, toothache, gnathological problems, teeth grinding.
J. Bischko: Peroral skin rash eruptions.

Action in TCM: Expels Wind, removes obstructions from the meridian, opens the mouth.

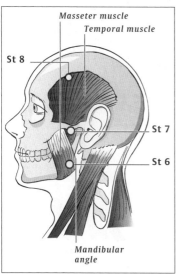

Masseter muscle
Temporal muscle

St 8

St 7

St 6

Mandibular angle

○ **St 7 "Xia Guan"**
"Lower Gate" ("Lower Pass")

Location: In the center of the depression below the zygomatic arch, i.e., in the mandibular notch between the coronoid process and the condylar process of mandible. The condylar process of mandible can be easily palpated in front of the tragus (it glides toward the front when the mouth is opened). Point St 7 lies in a depression right in front of it. This point is searched for and needled while the mouth is closed.

!

The lateral pterygoid muscle is reached by deep needling. With regard to its localization, Point St 7 often corresponds to a trigger point in the masseter muscle or in the lateral pterygoid muscle.

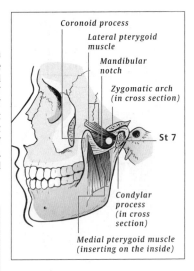

Coronoid process

Lateral pterygoid muscle

Mandibular notch

Zygomatic arch (in cross section)

St 7

Condylar process (in cross section)

Medial pterygoid muscle (inserting on the inside)

Depth of needling: 0.3 to 0.5 Cun, perpendicularly.

Indication: Myofacial pain dysfunction (Costen's syndrome), atypical facial pain, temporomandibular joint problems, facial paralysis, tinnitus, otalgia.

Action in TCM: Removes obstructions from the meridian, benefits the ear.
St 7 + St 44: Toothache in the upper jaw.

○ **St 8 "Tou Wei"**
"Head Support" ("Head Corner")

Location: 0.5 Cun into the hair from the frontal hairline, in the angle of this hairline with the temporal hairline running perpendicular to it. Hence, Point St 8 lies 4.5 Cun lateral to Point GV 24.

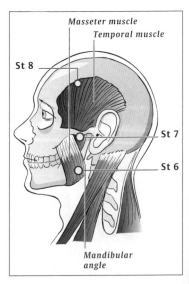

Masseter muscle

Temporal muscle

St 8

St 7

St 6

Mandibular angle

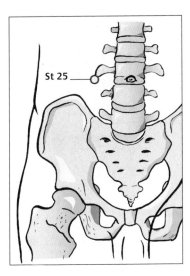

St 25

! Points St 6, 7, and 8 lie roughly on a vertical line. If the original frontal hairline can no longer be found because of hair loss, it can be found by frowning and identifying the border of the frontal folds.

Depth of needling: 2 to 4 mm, subcutaneously in dorsal direction.

Indication: Cephalalgia, migraine, eye disorders, atypical facial pain, vertigo.

Action in TCM: Expels exterior Wind, clears Heat, eliminates stagnation in the Large Intestine, transforms Dampness.

○ St 25 "Tian Shu"
   "Heavenly Pivot" ("Upper Pivot")
   Front Collecting Point (Mu Point) of
   the Large Intestine

Location: 2 Cun lateral to the navel.

Depth of needling: 0.5 to 1.5 Cun, perpendicularly.

Indication: Obstipation, meteorism, diarrhea, ulcers of the stomach and duodenum, Crohn's disease, ulcerative colitis, functional gastrointestinal problems.

Action in TCM: Promotes the circulation of Qi, cools Heat, eliminates stagnation in the Large Intestine, transforms Dampness.

○ **St 34 "Liang Qiu"**
"Beam Mound" ("Hill Ridge")
Cleft Point (Xi Point)

Location: With the knee slightly flexed, 2 Cun above the lateral upper margin of the patella, in a depression within the lateral vastus muscle. The point lies on the line connecting the superior anterior iliac spine and the lateral upper pole of the patella.

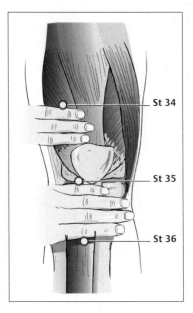

St 34

St 35

St 36

> **!** All points of the knee region are searched for and needled with the knee slightly flexed (use support padding to position the patient better).

Depth of needling: 1 to 2 Cun, perpendicularly.

Indication: Acute symptoms of the gastrointestinal tract, knee problems, nausea and vomiting; distal point used in mastitis.

Action in TCM: Removes obstructions from the meridian, subdues the rebellious Qi, expels Wind, Dampness, and Cold.

○ **St 35 "Du Bi"**
"Calf Nose"

Location: With the knee slightly flexed, below the patella and lateral to the patellar tendon, the lateral Knee Eye (the term Knee Eye applies to three points caudal, medial, and lateral to the patella). Thus, the lateral Knee Eye corresponds to Point St 35, the medial Knee Eye corresponds to Extra Point Xi Yan (EX-LE 5).

> **!** Do not needle too deeply because of the risk of positioning the needle intra-articularly. The lateral Knee Eye corresponds roughly to the localization of the arthroscopic access to the knee joint.

Depth of needling: 3 to 6 mm, in slightly oblique medial direction.

Indication: Gonalgia.

Action in TCM: Removes obstructions from the meridian, reduces swelling and pain, expels Wind, Dampness, and Cold.

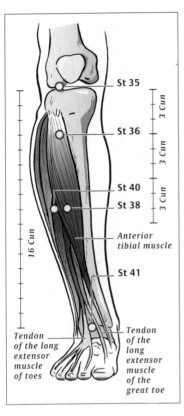

St 35

St 36

3 Cun

St 40

St 38

3 Cun

3 Cun

Anterior
tibial muscle

16 Cun

St 41

Tendon
of the long
extensor
muscle
of toes

Tendon
of the
long
extensor
muscle
of the
great toe

○ **St 36 "Zu San Li"**
"Three Miles of the Foot"
("Foot Three Li")
**Lower Sea Point (Lower He Point) of
the Stomach**

Location: With the knee slightly flexed, 3 Cun below Point St 35, roughly at the level of the lower border of the tibial tuberosity as well as about 1 Cun lateral to the tibial edge in the anterior tibial muscle.

!

● With dynamic palpating, a distinct depression is palpable at Point St 36. In the European literature, the distance is usually given as 1 Cun lateral to the tibial edge, while the Chinese literature always gives the slightly lesser width of 1 middle finger.

Depth of needling: 0.5 to 1.5 Cun, perpendicularly.

Indication: One of the most versatile and most often used acupuncture points (second to Point LI 4); a general tonification point often used in combination with moxa; homeostatic effect on metabolic diseases; distal point used in abdominal disorders; strongly harmonizing effect on the psyche.

Action in TCM: Strengthens Spleen and Stomach, tonifies Qi and Blood, regulates the circulation of Qi and Blood, strengthens Food Qi (Gu Qi) and Defensive Qi (Wei Qi), removes Dampness, dispels exterior pathogenic Cold, regulates the ascending pure Qi and the descending turbid Qi, calms the rebellious Qi, regulates the Intestines, stabilizes the Mind (Shen) and emotions.
St 36 + Lu 9: Qi Deficiency.

○ **St 38 "Tiao Kou"**
"Narrow Opening"
("Narrow Mouth")

Location: In the middle of the line connecting Points St 35 and St 41, one width of the middle finger lateral to the tibial edge, or 2 Cun caudal to St 37.

❗ According to *König and Wancura,* the middle is best determined using the hand-spreading method. For this purpose, the two little fingers are placed on Points St 35 and St 41 and the center is determined using both thumbs.

Depth of needling: 1 to 2 Cun, perpendicularly.

Indication: Distal point used in acute shoulder–arm syndrome.

Action in TCM: Removes obstructions from the meridian, relaxes the tendons, expels Cold.

○ **St 40 "Feng Long"**
"Abundant Bulge"
("Rich and Prosperous")
Connecting Point (Luo Point)

Location: 1 width of the middle finger lateral to Point St 38.

Depth of needling: 1 to 2 Cun, obliquely in medial direction.

Indication: Gastrointestinal disorders, hypersalivation (moisture), "mucous disorders," i.e., all diseases with excessive mucus production (mucous cough, mucous vomiting, mucous diarrhea).

Action in TCM: Transforms Phlegm and removes Dampness, stimulates the descending of turbid Qi, clears the Mind (Shen), regulates the circulation of Spleen Qi and Stomach Qi, opens the chest and calms asthma.

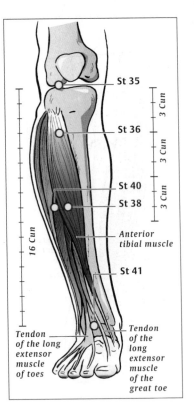

St 35

St 36

3 Cun

St 40

3 Cun

St 38

3 Cun

Anterior tibial muscle

16 Cun

St 41

Tendon of the long extensor muscle of toes

Tendon of the long extensor muscle of the great toe

> The tendon of the long extensor muscle of great toe can be recognized when the great toe is lifted; lateral to it is Point St 41.

Depth of needling: 0.5 to 1 Cun, perpendicularly.

Indication: Stomach problems, affections of the ankle joint.

Action in TCM: Calms the Mind, invigorates the Spleen.

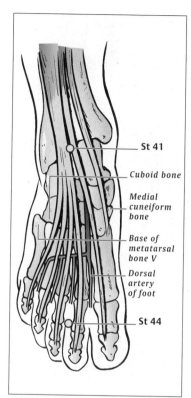

- St 41
- Cuboid bone
- Medial cuneiform bone
- Base of metatarsal bone V
- Dorsal artery of foot
- St 44

○ **St 41 "Jie Xi"**
"Dispersing Stream"
("Opened Hollow")
Tonification Point

Location: In the anterior middle of the line connecting the lateral malleolus with the medial malleolus, between the tendons of the long extensor muscle of great toe and the long extensor muscle of the toes over the upper ankle joint.

○ **St 44 "Nei Ting"**
"Inner Courtyard" ("Inner Court")

Location: At the end of the interdigital fold between second and third toes.

Depth of needling: 0.3 to 1 Cun, perpendicularly.

Indication: An important pain point; frontal headache, nose bleeding, feverish colds.
H. Schmidt: Effective against upset stomach.

Action in TCM: Cools Stomach Fire and Heat, relieves pain along the Stomach Meridian, removes Wind from the face, stimulates the descending of turbid Qi, regulates ascending Qi, harmonizes the flow of Qi in Stomach and Intestines.
St 44 + LI 4: Expel exterior and interior Wind (headache, facial pain, facial paresis, trigeminal neuralgia).

Major Points of the Spleen Meridian

Sp 3: Source Point (Yuan Point).
Sp 4: Connecting Point (Luo Point). Opening Point of the extraordinary meridian, Chong Mai (Penetrating Vessel).
Sp 6: Crossing Point of the three Yin Meridians of the foot.
Sp 9: Local point with remote effect.
Sp 10: Local point with remote effect.

Points Associated with the Spleen Meridian

Liv 13: Front Collecting Point (Mu Point) of the Spleen.
B 20: Back Transporting Point (Back Shu Point) of the Spleen.

Coupling Relationships of the Spleen Meridian

Top-to-bottom coupling:
Lung–Spleen

Yin-Yang coupling:
Spleen–Stomach

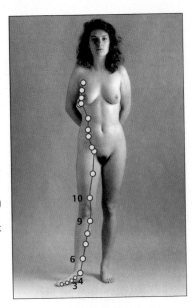

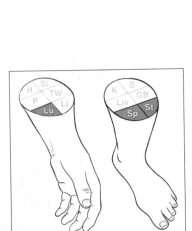

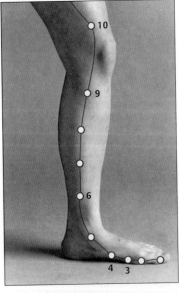

● **Sp 3 "Tai Bai"**
  "Greater White" ("Grand White,"
  "Supreme Whiteness")
  Source Point (Yuan Point)

Location: Inside of the foot, proximal to the head of metatarsal bone I, at the body–head transition of metatarsal bone I, at the border between red and white skin.

Depth of needling: 3 to 6 mm, perpendicularly.

Indication: General abdominal problems, lack of appetite, gastritis, vomiting, obstipation, diarrhea, meteorism, vertigo, chronic fatigue, sensation of fullness, and tension in the thorax and epigastric region.

Action in TCM: Important point for strengthening the Spleen Meridian; syndromes of Spleen Deficiency; harmonizes the flow of Qi in the Middle Warmer; important point in diseases of Dampness and Phlegm, in Bi syndromes with Cold, Heat, and Dampness; transforms Dampness, Damp Heat, and Phlegm.

Sp 3 + St 36: An important combination for tonifying Spleen and Qi.

Sp 3 + St 40: Eliminates Dampness and Phlegm.

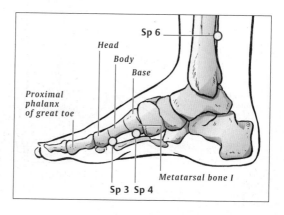

○ Sp 4 "Gong Sun"
"Minute Connecting Channels"
("Collateral Point of Spleen Channel,"
"Grandfather Grandson")
Connecting Point (Luo Point)
Opening Point of the Extraordinary
Meridian, Chong Mai
(Penetrating Vessel)

Location: In a depression at the body–base transition of metacarpal bone I, at the border between red and white skin.

Depth of needling: 0.5 to 1 Cun, perpendicularly.

Indication: Stomach problems, gastrocardiac syndrome, loss of appetite, indigestion with thin bowel movements, dysmenorrhea.
J. Bischko: Master Point for diarrhea.

Action in TCM: Tonifies Spleen and Stomach; regulates the flow of Qi in the Middle Warmer; mobilizes Qi and Blood; removes stagnation; regulates the Penetrating Vessel (Chong Mai); circulates Qi and Blood, especially in the Lower Warmer; subdues the rebellious Stomach Qi; stops bleeding; regulates menstruation.

Sp 4 + P 6 + CV 12: Abdominal problems, nausea, vomiting.

Sp 4 + St 36 + Sp 10: Stagnation of Blood.

Sp 4 + R 6 + CV 3: Stagnation of Qi and Blood, dysmenorrhea, difficult menstruation.

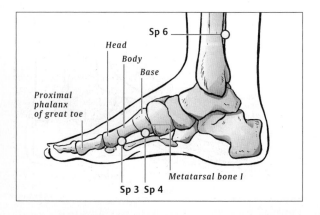

Sp 6

Head

Body

Base

Proximal
phalanx
of great toe

Metatarsal bone I

Sp 3   Sp 4

● **Sp 6 "San Yin Jiao"**
"Three Yin Meeting"
("Crossroad of Three Yins")
Crossing Point of the Three Yin
Meridians of the Foot

Location: 3 Cun above the largest prominence of the medial malleolus at the posterior tibial edge, in a depression often clearly palpable (particularly in women).

Occasionally, the point may be located slightly more to the front, i.e., in the tibial region.

Depth of needling: 1 to 2 Cun, perpendicularly.

Indication: The third most common acupuncture point; a general tonification point (moxa); "Royal Point" for all gynecological problems; facilitation of birth; acceleration of uterine contractions, gastrointestinal disorders, urogenital disorders (impotence, frigidity, dysmenorrhea); also effective in allergic and immunological diseases, skin disorders.

König and Wancura: Basic point in combination with Point H 7 when treating psychosomatic diseases.

Basic point in combination with Point CV 4 in disorders of the urogenital tract.

Caution! This point increases uterine contractions; therefore, it should not be needled during pregnancy.

Action in TCM: Nourishes particularly the Yin, tonifies Spleen and Blood, circulates Qi and Blood, eliminates stagnation of Blood and alleviates pain along the Lower Warmer; regulates the uterus and menstruation; eliminates stagnation in the Liver, calms ascending Liver Yang, tonifies Liver Yin and Liver Blood, removes Dampness particularly in the Lower Warmer, cools Blood Heat, tonifies the Kidney, calms the Mind (Shen) especially in the case of Blood Heat and Yin Deficiency.

Sp 6 + Sp 9: Eliminates Dampness.

Sp 6 + CV 12: Supports the digestive system.

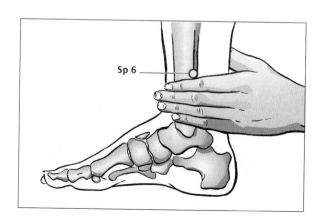

Sp 6

○ **Sp 9 "Yin Ling Quan"**
  "Yin Mound Spring"
  ("Yin Hill Fountain")

Location: In the depression distal to the medial condyle of tibia at the transition of the medial condyle of tibia–body of tibia, in front of the belly of the gastrocnemius muscle (at the same level as Point GB 34).

Depth of needling: 0.5 to 1 Cun, perpendicularly.

Indication: Main point for eliminating accumulations of water and moisture, especially in the lower half of the body, difficulties in passing urine, dysuria, infections of the urinary tract, dysmenorrhea, vaginal discharge, fetid diarrhea, abdominal spasm, gonalgia, arthritis of the knee joints.
H. Schmidt: Enuresis (moxa).

Action in TCM: The most important point for removing Dampness and Moisture; eliminates Damp Heat and Damp Cold, regulates the urinary tract and promotes the passing of urine, benefits the Lower Warmer, removes obstructions from the meridian.
Sp 9 + St 40: Dampness and Phlegm.
Sp 9 + P 6: Damp Heat in the Lower Warmer, vaginal discharge, cystitis.

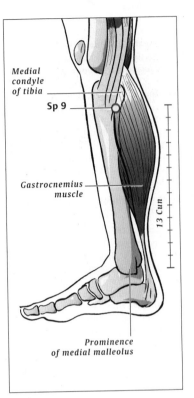

Medial condyle of tibia

Sp 9

Gastrocnemius muscle

13 Cun

Prominence of medial malleolus

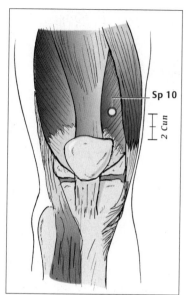

● Sp 10 "Xue Hai"
"Sea of Blood" ("Blood Sea")

Location: With the knee flexed, 2 Cun proximal to the medial cranial pole of the patella, on the medial vastus muscle in an often clearly palpable depression. Another possible localization: When placing the palm onto the patella with the thumb slightly spread, Point Sp 10 lies in front of the tip of the thumb.

Depth of needling: 1 to 2 Cun, perpendicularly.

Indication: An important immunomodulating point (together with Point LI 11). Skin disorders, pruritus, disorders of the urogenital tract, dysmenorrhea.

Action in TCM: An important point for regulating Blood; cools Blood, circulates Blood, removes stagnation, tonifies Blood, regulates menstruation.

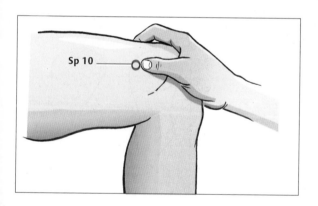

Major Points of the Heart Meridian

H 3:   Local point with general effect.
H 5:   Connecting Point (Luo Point).
H 7:   Source Point (Yuan Point). Sedation point.

Points Associated with the Heart Meridian

CV 14: Front Collecting Point (Mu Point) of the Heart.
B 15:   Back Transporting Point (Back Shu Point) of the Heart.

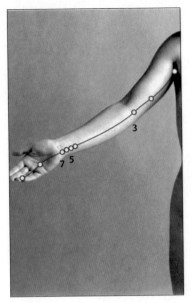

Coupling Relationships of the Heart Meridian

Top-to-bottom coupling:
Heart–Kidney

Yin-Yang coupling:
Heart–Small Intestine

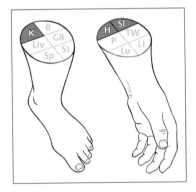

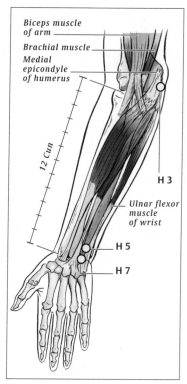

Biceps muscle
of arm

Brachial muscle
Medial
epicondyle
of humerus

12 Cun

H 3

Ulnar flexor
muscle
of wrist

H 5

H 7

◉ H 3 "Shao Hai"
"Lesser Yin Sea" ("Young Sea")

Location: When the elbow is flexed, the point lies between the ulnar end of the elbow flexion crease and the medial epicondyle of humerus.

Depth of needling: 0.5 to 1 Cun, perpendicularly.

Indication: "The Joy of Life," psychovegetative dysregulation, insomnia, mental agitation (Heart Fire, use sedative stimulation during the acute phase), depressive mood (caution when using the sedation method), vertigo, medial humeral epicondylitis (golfer's elbow), tremor of hands.

Action in TCM: Clears Heat from Heart and Pericardium (Full Fire or Empty Fire), clears and calms the Mind (Shen), removes obstructions from the meridian.

◉ H 5 "Tong Li"
"Inner Communication"
Connecting Point (Luo Point)

Location: 1 Cun proximal to Point H 7, radial to the tendon of the ulnar flexor muscle of wrist.

Depth of needling: Up to 0.5 Cun, perpendicularly.

Indication: Psychovegetative dysregulation, functional heart problems, fear of examinations, anxiety attacks and restlessness, insomnia, sweating.

Action in TCM: Main point for supporting the regulation of Heart Qi; cools Heart Heat, reveals itself in the tongue, regulates tongue and communication, calms the Mind (Shen).

○ **H 7 "Shen Men"**
"Mind Door" ("Spiritual Gate")
Source Point (Yuan Point)
Sedation Point

Location: At the flexion crease of the wrist, radial to the tendon of the ulnar flexor muscle of wrist.

> ❗ The flexion crease required for its localization lies between the radius and ulna on the one side and the bones of the wrist on the other. This region is clearly marked in ulnar direction by the pisiform bone. Hence, the flexion crease of the wrist lying proximal to the pisiform bone is used.

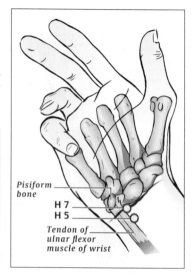

Pisiform bone
H 7
H 5
Tendon of ulnar flexor muscle of wrist

According to many descriptions in the German literature, a second possibility for needling is from the ulnar side. The direction of needling is here parallel to the flexion crease of the wrist, i.e., at an angle of 90° relative to the needling method first described. The tip of the needle then lies dorsal to the tendon of the ulnar flexor muscle of wrist. Point H 7 lies deep where the tips of the two needles would meet if coming from volar and ulnar directions. This direction of needling, however, is not known in the Chinese literature.

Depth of needling: 0.3 to 0.5 Cun, perpendicularly, from volar or ulnar direction.

Indication: Insomnia, anxiety attacks, circulatory dysregulation, withdrawal symptoms during addiction therapy, hyperactivity.
König and Wancura: In combination with Point Sp 6, it is the backbone for the treatment of psychosomatic disorders.

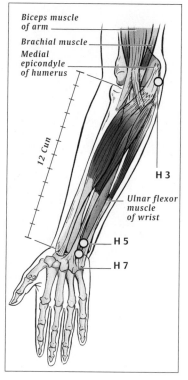

Biceps muscle
of arm

Brachial muscle

Medial
epicondyle
of humerus

12 Cun

H 3

Ulnar flexor
muscle
of wrist

H 5

H 7

Action in TCM: When using the sedation method: cools Heart Fire and Heart Heat, eliminates stagnation of Qi, Blood, and Phlegm in the Heart Meridian, calms the Mind (Shen).

When using the tonification method: nourishes Heart Blood, Qi, and Yin.

!

● Consider stimulation; sedate Point H 7 only in case of confirmed syndromes of Excess; watch for red tip of the tongue (e.g., Heart Heat)!

H 7 + P 7: Nervous conditions of anxiety and tension.

Major Points of the Small Intestine Meridian

SI 3: Tonification point. Opening Point of the Governor Vessel, Du Mai.
SI 8: Sedation point.
SI 11: Local point.
SI 12: Local point.
SI 14: Local point.
SI 18: Local point.
SI 19: Local point.

Points Associated with the Small Intestine Meridian

CV 4: Front Collecting Point (Mu Point) of the Small Intestine.
B 27: Back Transporting Point (Back Shu Point) of the Small Intestine.
St 39: Lower Sea Point (Lower He Point) of the Small Intestine.

Coupling Relationships of the Small Intestine Meridian

Top-to-bottom coupling:
Small Intestine–Bladder

Yin-Yang coupling:
Small Intestine–Heart

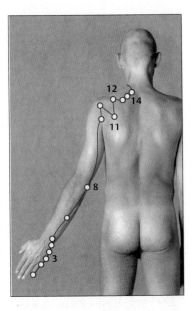

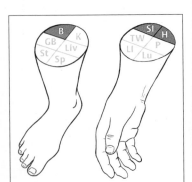

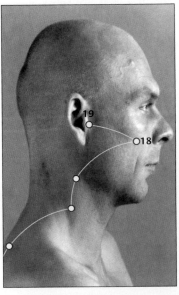

○ **SI 3 "Hou Xi"**
"Back Stream"
Tonification Point
Opening Point of the Governor
Vessel, Du Mai

Location: At the ulnar edge of the hand, with the fist lightly closed, proximal and dorsal to a skin fold at the ulnar end of the most distal flexion crease of the palm. The point is located at the body–head transition of metacarpal bone V (*Gleditsch, König and Wancura*).

> ❗ With the fist lightly closed, the distal flexion crease of the palm is followed in ulnar direction. It usually starts between index and middle fingers. At the end of the flexion crease there is a small bulge of the skin. At the border of this bulge to the surrounding area, slightly proximal and dorsal, lies Point SI 3. The needle is directed toward the middle of the palm.

According to Chinese literature, the point is localized at the distal end of the flexion crease described, at the transition from red to white skin. Needling takes place in vertical direction. With the localization given above, however, needling takes place in a slightly distal direction. Hence, the slightly different localizations of this point meet deep where the De Qi sensation originates. In our experience, the localization given by *Gleditsch*, which is also described by *König and Wancura*, proved more effective in both diagnosis and therapy.

Depth of needling: 0.5 to 1 Cun in the direction of the palm.

Indication: Acute lumbar pain, lumbago–sciatica syndrome; distal point for the cervical spine; torticollis, paresis of the upper extremity, tinnitus, hearing difficulty, diseases of the ear, feverish colds, pharyngitis, laryngitis, tremor, vertigo.

J. Bischko: The main indication for this point is spasmolysis.

Advice: In acute torticollis, acute lumbago, or lumbago–sciatica syndrome, treatment is followed by vigorous stimulation of Point SI 3 while simultaneously cautiously undertaking physical exercise.

Action in TCM: Opens the Governor Vessel, expels exterior pathogenic factors, especially Wind and Heat, eliminates interior Wind from the Governor Vessel, removes obstructions from the meridian and collateral vessels, relaxes muscles and tendons, clears and calms the Mind (Shen).

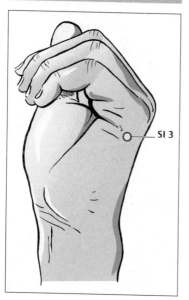

SI 3

○ **SI 8 "Xiao Hai"**
 "Small Intestine Sea" ("Small Sea")
 Sedation Point

Location: When the arm is flexed, in the ulnar sulcus between the olecranon and medial epicondyle of humerus.

Depth of needling: 4 to 8 mm, perpendicularly.
Advice: Point SI 8 lies in close proximity to the ulnar nerve which might be accidentally needled; in this case, withdraw the needle immediately but do not remove it completely.

Indication: Medial humeral epicondylitis (golfer's elbow); pain in the throat, shoulder, and neck regions.

Action in TCM: Removes obstructions from the meridian, removes Dampness and Heat.

○ **SI 11 "Tian Zong"**
 "Heavenly Attribution"
 ("Celestial Watching")

Location: In the infraspinous fossa on a line connecting the middle of the clearly palpable scapular spine and the inferior angle of scapula. Point SI 11 lies on this line between the cranial third and the remaining two-thirds. It lies immediately below Point SI 12 at the level of the lower edge of the spinous process of T4 and forms a triangle with Points SI 9 and SI 10 (see fig. on p. 37).

Depth of needling: 0.5 to 1 Cun, perpendicularly.

Indication: Pain and loss of motion in the shoulder (especially on exterior rotation), tightness in the thorax; in combination with other points in cases of difficult lactation and mastitis.
H. Schmidt: Special point for insufficient lactation.

Action in TCM: Removes obstructions from the meridian, expels exterior pathogen factors from the Tai Yang Meridians (SI and B).
SI 11 + SI 1 + St 18: Difficult lactation and mastitis.

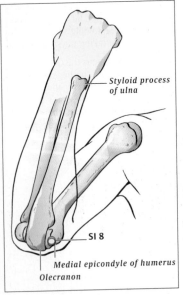

Styloid process of ulna

SI 8

Medial epicondyle of humerus
Olecranon

○ SI 12 "Bing Feng"
  "Watching Wind"

Location: Perpendicularly above Point SI 11, approximately 1 Cun above the middle of the cranial border of the scapular spine. The point forms a triangle with Points SI 10 and SI 11. Common trigger point in the supraspinous muscle.

Depth of needling: 0.5 to 1 Cun, perpendicularly.

Indication: Pain and loss of motion in the shoulder (especially on abduction and exterior rotation), supraspinatus syndrome, pain and paresthesia of the upper extremity, stiff neck.

Action in TCM: Removes obstructions from the meridian and collateral vessels.

○ SI 14 "Jian Wai Shu"
  "Transporting Point of the Outside of the Shoulder"
  ("Exterior Shoulder")

Location: 3 Cun lateral to the spinous process of T1.
Common trigger point in the levator muscle of scapula.

❗ When the patient's arms are hanging down, the distance between the dorsal median line and the medial end of scapular spine is 3 Cun.

Depth of needling: 0.5 to 1 Cun, perpendicularly.

Indication: Pain and loss of motion in the shoulder, stiff neck.

Action in TCM: Removes obstructions from the meridian, purges Wind and Cold.

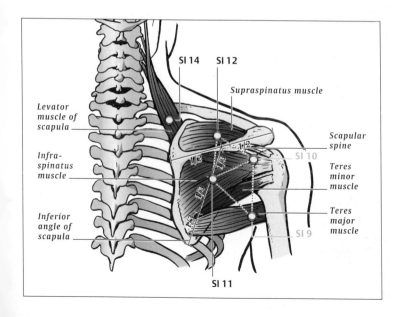

○ **SI 18 "Quan Liao"**
"Zygoma Crevice" ("Cheek Crevice")

Location: At the lower edge of the zygomatic arch, perpendicularly below the outer corner of the eye, at the anterior margin of the masseter muscle.

> **!** The anterior margin of the masseter muscle is clearly palpable during chewing.

Depth of needling: 0.3 to 0.5 Cun, perpendicularly.

Indication: Myofacial pain dysfunction (Costen's syndrome), trigeminal neuralgia, facial spasm, facial paresis, toothache, maxillary sinusitis, gnathological problems.

Action in TCM: Important point in facial disorders of Wind Cold and Wind Heat; relieves pain.

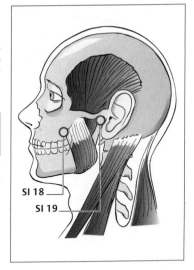

SI 18

SI 19

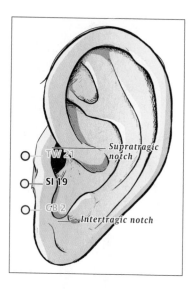

○ **SI 19 "Ting Gong"**
   "Listening Palace"

Location: In the depression in front of the tragus.

> **!**
> Localization takes place with the mouth slightly opened; this way, the condylar process of mandible of the temporomandibular joint moves in nasal direction so that there is no risk of needling the temporomandibular joint. The mouth is closed after inserting the needle.
> Advice: Point SI 19 lies in close proximity of the superficial temporal artery which can be avoided by palpating its pulse prior to needling.

Depth of needling: 0.3 to 0.5 Cun, perpendicularly.

Indication: Ear disorders, facial paresis, trigeminal neuralgia, myofacial pain dysfunction (Costen's syndrome), temporomandibular joint dysfunction.

Action in TCM: Opens and supports the ear.

Major Points of the Bladder Meridian

B 2: Local point.

B 10: Point with an influence on the parasympathetic nervous system.

B 11: Master Point of the bones.

B 13: Back Shu Point of the Lung.

B 14: Back Shu Point of the Pericardium.

B 15: Back Shu Point of the Heart.

B 17: Back Shu Point of the diaphragm. Master Point of the blood.

B 18: Back Shu Point of the Liver.

B 19: Back Shu Point of the Gall Bladder.

B 20: Back Shu Point of the Spleen.

B 21: Back Shu Point of the Stomach.

B 23: Back Shu Point of the Kidney.

B 25: Back Shu Point of the Large Intestine.

B 27: Back Shu Point of the Small Intestine.

B 28: Back Shu Point of the Bladder.

B 36: Local point with a wide spectrum of activity.

B 40: Lower Sea Point (Lower He Point) of the Bladder.

B 43: Point with a wide spectrum of activity.

B 54: Local point.

B 57: Local point.

B 60: Peripheral pain point.

B 62: Opening Point of the extraordinary meridian, Yang Qiao Mai (Yang Heel Vessel).

B 67: Tonification point.

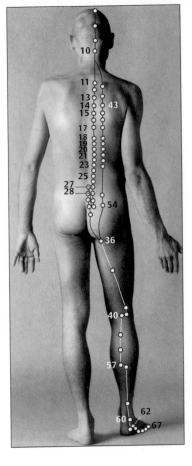

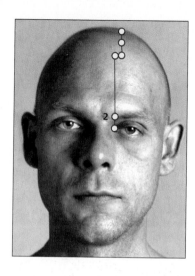

Points Associated with the Bladder Meridian

CV 3: Front Collecting Point (Mu Point) of the Bladder.

B 28: Back Transporting Point (Back Shu Point) of the Bladder.

B 40: Lower Sea Point (Lower He Point) of the Bladder.

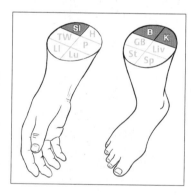

Coupling Relationships of the Bladder Meridian

Top-to-bottom coupling:
Small Intestine–Bladder

Yin-Yang coupling:
Bladder–Kidney

◎ B 2 "Zan Zhu"
"Collecting Bamboo"
("Gathering Eyebrows")

Location: At the medial end of the eyebrow, above the inner corner of the eye. The point is located over the often palpable medial frontal notch at the edge of the orbit.

> **!** The frontal notch represents the exit of the supratrochlear artery and the medial branch of the supraorbital nerve. It is not the supraorbital foramen, which is clearly further lateral and represents the exit of both the supraorbital artery and the lateral branch of the supraorbital nerve. Both points of exit vary in shape and position. The frontal notch rarely appears as frontal foramen; the supraorbital foramen rarely appears as supraorbital notch.

Advice: The Chinese literature mentions a "supraorbital notch" through which the medial branch of the supraorbital nerve passes. This notch does not represent the supraorbital foramen.

Depth of needling: Approx. 0.3 Cun, subcutaneously toward the root of the nose or caudally in the direction of Point B 1.

Indication: Eye disorders, cephalalgia, disorders of the nasal pharynx, pollinosis, the urge to sneeze, glaucoma, insufficient lacrimal secretion, vertigo, anosmia, tic, frontal sinusitis. Both B 2 Points (B 2 on the left and B 2 on the right) combined with the Extra Point Yin Tang (EX-HN 3) form the "ventral magic triangle." These three points combined have a strong effect on the nasal pharynx (see also EX-HN 3, p. 105).

Action in TCM: Expels exterior pathogenic factors, especially Wind and Heat, clears and strengthens the eyes, calms Liver and nourishes Wood, regulates lacrimal secretion, removes obstructions from the meridian.

◎ B 10 "Tian Zhu"
"Heavenly Pillar" ("Celestial Pillar")

Location: Vertical orientation: 1.3 Cun lateral to the median line (Governor Vessel), in the belly of the trapezius muscle (just at the point where it begins to descend). Point B 10 lies 0.5 Cun cranial to the dorsal hairline, lateral to Point GV 15, close to the exit of the greater occipital nerve.
Horizontal orientation: above the spinous process of C2 (axis).

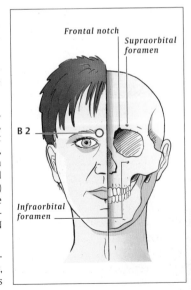

Frontal notch

Supraorbital foramen

B 2

Infraorbital foramen

!
  ● Point B 10 is located at the level between C1 (atlas) and C2 (axis). On palpation, this region lies cranial to the first palpable vertebral spinous process (the atlas does not have a spinous process). Palpation is usually better achieved when the head is slightly retroflexed to relax the often very tight nuchal ligament.

Remark: Point B 10 lies slightly more medial and caudal than Point GB 20.

Depth of needling: 0.5 to 1 Cun, perpendicularly.

!
  ● To eliminate any possibility of puncturing the spinal cord, especially in cachectic patients, the depth of needling should not exceed 1.5 Cun.

Indication: Strong effect on nose and eyes, enhancing effect on Point B 2 (front–back coupling), generalized vagus effect; anosmia, cervical syndrome, vertigo, migraine, colds, tonsillitis; affects the regulation of the body's overall tonus (see Point GB 20, p. 78).

Action in TCM: Expels exterior and interior Wind, disperses Cold, cools Heat, clears eyes, head, and brain, removes obstructions from the meridian, relaxes muscles and tendons, strengthens the lower back.

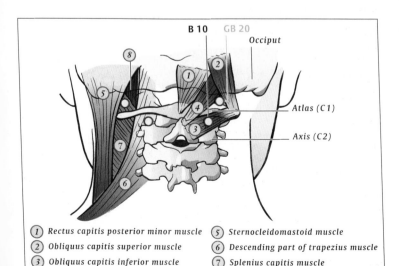

B 10   GB 20
Occiput
⑧
②
①
⑤
④ ─── Atlas (C1)
③ ─── Axis (C2)
⑦
⑥

① Rectus capitis posterior minor muscle
② Obliquus capitis superior muscle
③ Obliquus capitis inferior muscle
④ Rectus capitis posterior major muscle
⑤ Sternocleidomastoid muscle
⑥ Descending part of trapezius muscle
⑦ Splenius capitis muscle
⑧ Semispinalis capitis muscle

○ B 11 "Da Zhu"
"Big Reed" ("Great Axle")
Master Point of the Bones

Location: 1.5 Cun lateral to the lower edge of the spinous process of T1.

!
● When the arms are hanging down, the distance between median line and medial margin of scapula (at the level of the clearly palpable attachment of the scapular spine at the medial margin of scapula) is 3 Cun.
To make learning easier: The last digit in the numbering of Bladder Meridian Points B 11 and B 17 follows the numbering of the thoracic vertebrae (e.g., Point B 11 lies below T1, Point B 13 below T3).

Depth of needling: 0.5 Cun, perpendicularly or in oblique medial direction.
Advice: When needling in oblique medial direction, guide the tip of the needle in slight caudal direction.

Indication: Cervical syndrome, shoulder–arm syndrome, sinusitis, cephalalgia, bronchial asthma, feverish colds.

Action in TCM: Removes obstructions from the meridian, relaxes muscles and tendons, expels exterior pathogenic factors such as Wind and Heat, tonifies Blood.
B 11 (on both sides) + GV 14: The "dorsal magic triangle" has a relaxing and calming effect.

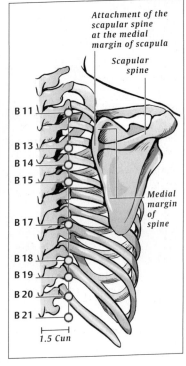

Attachment of the scapular spine at the medial margin of scapula

Scapular spine

B 11

B 13

B 14

B 15

B 17

Medial margin of spine

B 18

B 19

B 20

B 21

1.5 Cun

○ B 13 "Fei Shu"
  "Lung Back Transporting Point"
  ("Lung Shu")
  Back Shu Point of the Lung

Location: 1.5 Cun lateral to the lower edge of the spinous process of T3.

!
● In the standing patient with his/her arms hanging down, the lower edge of the spinous process of T3 is usually found at the level of the attachment of the clearly palpable scapular spine at the medial margin of scapula. As the Back Transporting Points are segmentally assigned to the organs of the functional circles, the Back Transporting Points of the thoracic organs (lungs, circulatory system, heart) lie in the thoracic region, those of the digestive organs (liver, spleen, pancreas, stomach) in the abdominal region, and those of the urogenital organs (kidney, bladder) in the lumbar region.

Depth of needling: 0.5 Cun, perpendicularly or obliquely.
Advice: When needling in oblique medial direction, guide the needle slightly in caudal direction to avoid any possibility of puncturing the spinal cord.

Indication: Disorders of the respiratory tract, asthma, cough, dyspnea, night sweat.

Action in TCM: Regulates and tonifies the Lung Qi, stimulates the dispersing and descending functions of the Lung, cools Heat and Empty Heat (Yin Deficiency) of the Lung, disperses the stagnation of Qi, eliminates Phlegm from the Lung; calms cough, sorrow, unresolved grief, and the clinging to the past.

○ B 14 "Jue Yin Shu"
  "Jue Yin Back Transporting Point"
  ("Pericardium Shu")
  Back Shu Point of the Pericardium
  (Circulatory System—Sexuality)

Location: 1.5 Cun lateral to the lower edge of the spinous process of T4.

Depth of needling: 0.5 Cun, perpendicularly or in oblique medial–caudal direction (see Points B 11 and B 13).

Indication: Functional heart problems, singultus, psychosomatic problems, angina pectoris, bronchitis, bronchial asthma, circulatory dysregulation.

Action in TCM: Regulates the Heart, relaxes the chest.

● B 15 "Xin Shu"
"Heart Back Transporting Point"
("Heart Shu")
Back Shu Point of the Heart

Location: 1.5 Cun lateral to the lower edge of the spinous process of T5.

Depth of needling: 0.5 Cun, perpendicularly or in oblique medial–caudal direction (see Points B 11 and B 13).

Indication: Diseases of the heart, fever, night sweat, menopausal problems, insomnia, restlessness.
H. Schmidt: Use intracutaneous permanent needling in case of paroxysmal tachycardia; fear of examination.

Action in TCM: Clears Heat, calms the Mind (Shen), stimulates the brain, invigorates Blood, nourishes Heart.
B 13 + LI 11: Pruritus (Blood Heat).

● B 17 "Ge Shu"
"Diaphragm Back Transporting Point"
("Diaphragm Shu")
Back Shu Point of the Diaphragm
Master Point of the Blood

Location: 1.5 Cun lateral to the lower edge of the spinous process of T7.

! In the standing patient with his/her arms hanging down, the lower edge of T7 is usually found at the level of the inferior angle of scapula.

Depth of needling: 0.5 Cun, perpendicularly or in oblique medial–caudal direction (see Points B 11 and B 13).

Indication: Prominent effect on the diaphragm; singultus, gastrocardiac syndrome, vomiting, bronchial asthma, hematological disorders with a venous component, dyspnea, urticaria.

Action in TCM: Nourishes and regulates Blood, removes stagnation of Blood, cools Blood Heat, relaxes chest and diaphragm, tonifies Blood and Qi, harmonizes Stomach Qi.

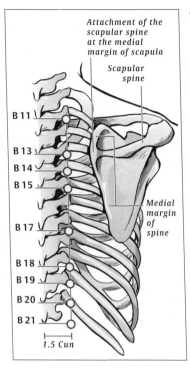

Attachment of the scapular spine at the medial margin of scapula

Scapular spine

B 11

B 13

B 14

B 15

B 17

Medial margin of spine

B 18

B 19

B 20

B 21

1.5 Cun

○ **B 18 "Gan Shu"**
"Liver Back Transporting Point"
("Liver Shu")
Back Shu Point of the Liver

Location: 1.5 Cun lateral to the lower edge of the spinous process of T9.

! To make learning easier: Up to Point B 17, the last digit in the numbering of Bladder Meridian Points follows the numbering of the thoracic vertebrae (e.g., Point B 17 lies below T7); starting with Point B 18, one vertebra is added (e.g. Point B 18 lies below T9).

Depth of needling: 0.5 Cun, perpendicularly or in oblique medial–caudal direction (see Points B 11 and B 13).

Indication: Disturbed liver metabolism, disturbed vision, vertigo, tension in the epigastric region and hypochondriac region, difficult menstruation, muscular tension, muscular cramps, pain in the upper abdomen, emotional hyperexcitability.

Action in TCM: Regulates and tonifies Liver and Gall Bladder, nourishes Liver Blood, removes stagnation of Liver Qi, calms interior Wind, cools Damp Heat in Liver and Gall Bladder, benefits the eyes.

○ **B 19 "Dan Shu"**
"Gall Bladder Back Transporting Point" ("Gall Bladder Shu")
Back Shu Point of the Gall Bladder

Location: 1.5 Cun lateral to the lower edge of the spinous process of T10.

Depth of needling: 0.5 Cun, perpendicularly or in oblique medial–caudal direction (see Points B 11 and B 13).

Indication: Disorders of the gall bladder, vomiting, bitter taste in the mouth, acid reflux.

Action in TCM: Regulates Gall Bladder, supports the eyes, cools Damp Heat in Liver and Gall Bladder, relaxes diaphragm and chest, harmonizes Stomach Qi.

○ **B 20 "Pi Shu"**
"Spleen Back Transporting Point" ("Spleen Shu")
Back Shu Point of the Spleen

Location: 1.5 Cun lateral to the lower edge of the spinous process of T11.

Depth of needling: 0.5 Cun, perpendicularly or in oblique medial–caudal direction (see Points B 11 and B 13).

Indication: Important point for treating the gastrointestinal tract; meteorism, dysentery, loss of appetite, ulcers of stomach and duodenum, abdominal sensation of tension and fullness, diarrhea, edematous swellings, chronic mucus diseases of the respiratory tract, convalescence.

Action in TCM: Important point for all syndromes of Spleen Emptiness, tonifies Spleen and Stomach, nourishes Blood, removes Dampness, transforms Phlegm.
B 20 + B 21: General tonification of Qi and Blood.

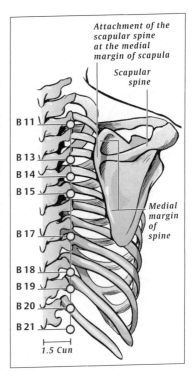

Attachment of the scapular spine at the medial margin of scapula

Scapular spine

B 11
B 13
B 14
B 15
B 17
B 18
B 19
B 20
B 21

Medial margin of spine

1.5 Cun

● **B 21 "Wei Shu"**
"Stomach Back Transporting Point"
"Stomach Shu"
Back Shu Point of the Stomach

Location: 1.5 Cun lateral to the lower edge of the spinous process of T12.

Depth of needling: 0.5 Cun, perpendicularly or in oblique medial–caudal direction.

Indication: Disorders of the stomach, digestive problems, nausea, vomiting, disturbed gastric motility, singultus, loss of appetite.

Action in TCM: Important point for tonifying and regulating the Stomach, harmonizes and descends Stomach Qi, removes Dampness and Food stagnation.

● **B 23 "Shen Shu"**
"Kidney Back Transporting Point"
("Kidney Shu," "Sea of Vitality")
Back Shu Point of the Kidney

Location: 1.5 Cun lateral to the lower edge of the spinous process of L2.

! For locating vertebra L2, it is recommended to start at the iliac crest (vertebra L4, see Point B 25).

Depth of needling: 0.5 to 1.5 Cun, perpendicularly.

Indication: An excellent point for strengthening the renal function and circulation, used for all chronic diseases: chronic weakness and exhaustion, chronic lumbago, chronic asthma, disorders of the urogenital tract, allergies, rheumatic complaints. This point is among the major points often used with moxa.
J. Bischko: In cases where cold brings in a change for the worse.

Action in TCM: Tonifies the Kidney, strengthens the lower back, tonifies Kidney Yin and Kidney Yang (predominantly), nourishes Essence (Jing), nourishes Blood, supports the Bones and Marrow, strengthens hearing and vision, stimulates the Kidney's function of receiving Qi, removes Dampness.
B 23 + SI 4: Tonify Qi(moxa).

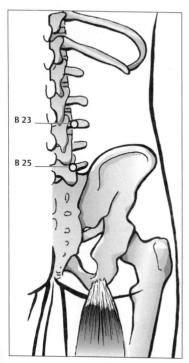

○ B 25 "Da Chang Shu"
"Large Intestine Back Transporting Point" ("Large Intestine Shu")
Back Shu Point of the Large Intestine

Location: 1.5 Cun lateral to the lower edge of the spinous process of L4.

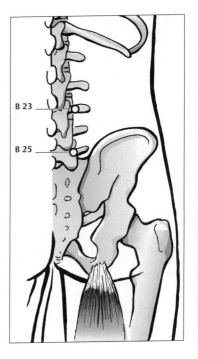

❗ Vertebra L4 is located at the level of the iliac crest (palpation from caudal to prevent skin folds from pressing on the iliac crest.) The lower edge of the spinous process lies a bit deeper.

Depth of needling: 0.5 to 1.5 Cun, perpendicularly.

Indication: Obstipation, diarrhea, disorders of the large intestine; important local point in cases of lumbago.

Action in TCM: Removes stagnation.

○ B 27 "Xiao Chang Shu"
"Small Intestine Back Transporting Point"
("Small Intestine Shu")
Back Shu Point of the Small Intestine

Location: At the level of the first sacral foramen, 1.5 Cun lateral to the dorsal median line, in a depression between sacrum and upper region of the superior posterior iliac spine.

❗ On palpation of the superior posterior iliac spine, Point B 27 is located in cranial and medial direction. Palpation of the superior posterior iliac spine is always performed from caudal because the bony pole is curved caudally. Aid in localizing the superior posterior iliac spine: starting at the gluteal cleft, palpate approximately 3 Cun at an angle of 45° in laterocranial direction.

Depth of needling: 0.5 to 1.5 Cun, perpendicularly; possibly in slightly oblique lateral direction toward the sacroiliac joint.

Indication: Lumbago, diseases of the genitals, spontaneous ejaculation, enuresis.

Action in TCM: Removes Dampness, regulates the urinary tract, removes stagnation.

B 28 "Pang Guang Shu"
"Bladder Back Transporting Point"
("Bladder Shu")
Back Shu Point of the Bladder

Location: At the level of the second sacral foramen, 1.5 Cun lateral to the dorsal median line. On palpation of the superior posterior iliac spine (see Point B 27), Point B 28 lies slightly caudal and medial.

Depth of needling: 0.5 to 1.5 Cun, perpendicularly; possibly in slightly oblique lateral direction toward the sacroiliac joint.

Indication: Lumbago, diseases of the bladder.

Action in TCM: Removes Dampness, regulates the urinary tract in the Lower Warmer, removes stagnation, eliminates Heat.

B 36 "Cheng Fu"
"Receiving Support"
("Supporting by Hand")

Location: In the middle of the gluteal crease (not of the femur).
Advice: This point lies in close proximity to the sciatic nerve. In case of deep needling, it is possible to puncture the nerve; the needle's position in the perineural tissue explains part of the acupuncture effect.

Depth of needling: 0.5 to 1.5 Cun, perpendicularly.

Indication: Lumbago–sciatica syndrome.

! Point B 36 lies over the ischial tuberosity. This point is also painful in enthesopathy of the ischiocrural muscles (semitendinous muscle, semimembranous muscle, biceps muscle of thigh).

Action in TCM: Removes stagnation.

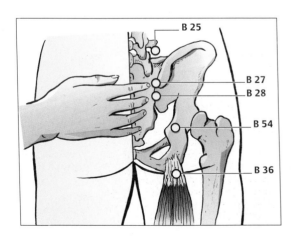

● B 40 "Wei Zhong"
  "Supporting Middle"
  ("Popliteal Center")
  Lower Sea Point (Lower He Point) of
  the Bladder

Location: In the middle of the popliteal cavity. This point lies close to the tibial nerve and the popliteal artery.

Depth of needling: 0.5 to 1 Cun, perpendicularly.

Indication: Lumbago, gonalgia, paresis of the lower extremity; an important distal point for the lower lumbar spine region; skin disorders, kidney and bladder diseases, eczema, herpes zoster, psoriasis (Blood Heat, use microphlebotomy), dysuria.
H. Schmidt: Microphlebotomy is often a good idea.

Action in TCM: Removes obstructions from the meridian and collateral vessels, relaxes the tendons, strengthens the lower back and the knee, clears Heat, removes Damp Heat, cools Blood, eliminates stagnation of Blood.
Advice: Use Point B 40 in conditions of congestion (Fullness); Point B 60 is better suited in chronic conditions (Emptiness) and symptoms of Cold.

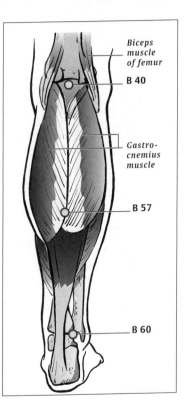

Biceps muscle of femur

B 40

Gastro-cnemius muscle

B 57

B 60

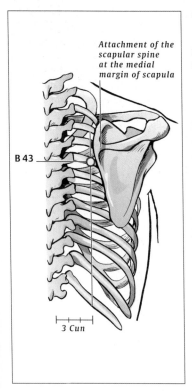

Attachment of the
scapular spine
at the medial
margin of scapula

B 43

3 Cun

B 43 "Gao Huang"
"Vitals" ("Vital Organs")

Location: 3 Cun lateral to the lower edge of the spinous process of T4.

!

● The localization of Point B 43 corresponds to a very frequent trigger point in the greater rhomboid muscle or in the iliocostal muscle of thorax. Upon deep needling, the tip of the needle passes through quite a few muscles (ascending part of trapezius muscle, greater rhomboid muscle, iliocostal muscle of thorax) which are innervated by the spinal nerves of various segments (C4–C5, T1–T4). The ascending part of the trapezius muscle developed embrologically from portions of the head mesenchyme and is innervated by the accessory nerve. Hence, the broad effect of Point B 43 covering several segments can also be explained in terms of conventional medicine.

Depth of needling: 0.5 to 1 Cun, subcutaneously in oblique direction toward Point B 14 (enhancing the effect), or 0.5 Cun in vertical direction, using the two-finger-protection method.

Indication: Diseases of the respiratory tract, insomnia, palpitation, loss of concentration, impotence, gastrointestinal disorders, back pain; broad spectrum of indications: this point is indicated in chronic disorders that are otherwise resistant to therapy.

Action in TCM: Tonifies Qi, nourishes Essence (Jing), nourishes Lung Yin, Kidney, and Heart, invigorates the Mind (Shen).

● B 54 "Zhi Bian"
"Lowermost Edge"
("Lowermost in Order")

Location: 3 Cun lateral to the sacral hiatus at the level of the fourth sacral foramen.

! When needling Point B 54, the gluteus maximus muscle and, still deeper, the piriformis muscle are reached. Here lie important trigger points of both these muscles. Tensions in both muscles play a major role in causing pain in the lumbar–pelvic–hip region. As the sciatic nerve lies in the depth, there is a risk of puncturing it by deep needling.

In about 20 % of cases, the sciatic nerve runs through the piriformis muscle. This is the case when the point of ramification lies high; the fibular part runs through the piriformis muscle while the tibial part runs through the infrapiriform foramen. This explains the irritation and cause of pain when the tonus of the piriformis muscle increases; hence, painfulness is not always the only cause of trigger points in this region.

Depth of needling: 1 to 2 Cun, perpendicularly.

Indication: Important distal point for lumbar spine problems (use deep needling); segmental relationship.

Action in TCM: Removes obstructions from the meridian and collateral vessels, relaxes the tendons, removes Dampness and Cold (very effective with moxa).

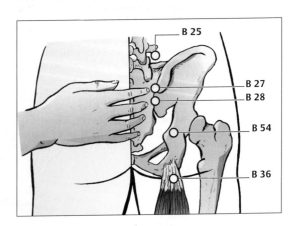

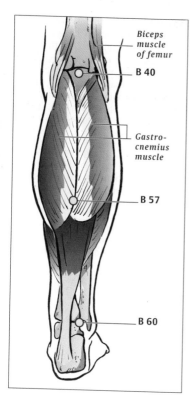

Biceps muscle of femur

B 40

Gastro-cnemius muscle

B 57

B 60

○ **B 57 "Cheng Shan"**
"Supporting Mountain"
("Supporting Hill")

Location: Halfway between Points B 40 and B 60; 8 Cun caudal to B 40 in a depression between the bellies of the gastrocnemius muscle.

!
● Standing on the toes clearly demonstrates the calf muscles (especially the gastrocnemius muscle)
Another way of localization is by means of the hand-spreading method: in the middle between Points B 40 and B 60. (For details of the method, see Point St 38.)

Depth of needling: 0.5 to 1 Cun, perpendicularly.

Indication: Sciatica-like problems, cramps in the calf muscles, pain in the Achilles tendon; important distal point for lumbar spine problems and for the anal region (hemorrhoids), peripheral circulation disorders (intermittent claudication).

Action in TCM: Removes obstructions from the meridian and collateral vessels, relaxes the tendons, clears Damp Heat, invigorates Blood.

○ B 60 "Kun Lun"
 "Kun Lun Mountains"
 ("Big and High")

Location: In the middle of the line connecting the lateral malleolus and Achilles tendon.

! The De Qi sensation often appears clearly when the needle is directed toward the calcaneus. Point B 60 is often described in the literature as lying opposite Point K 3. However, this is not the case as outer and inner ankle do not lie on the same level.

Depth of needling: 0.5 to 1 Cun, perpendicularly.

Indication: One of the major peripheral pain points, especially for the lower extremity. Pain syndromes of the spine, cephalalgia, pain in the Achilles tendon, affections in the region of the ankle joint, painful menstruation occurring during dysmenorrhea with dark, clotted menstrual blood, protracted course of child birth, placental retention.

Action in TCM: Invigorates renal function and circulation, strengthens back and knee, relaxes muscles and tendons, removes obstructions from the meridian and collateral vessels, clears Heat, distributes Blood and removes stagnation of Blood in the uterus, eliminates pathogenic factors from the Tai Yang axis, expels interior and exterior Wind.
Caution! Needling during pregnancy is contraindicated.

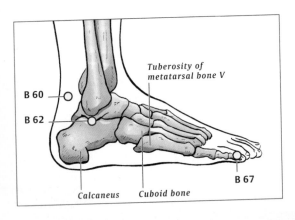

Tuberosity of metatarsal bone V

B 60

B 62

B 67

Calcaneus   *Cuboid bone*

○ B 62 "Shen Mai"
   "Ninth Channel"
   ("Stretching Channel")
   Opening Point of the Extraordinary
   Meridian, Yang Qiao Mai
   (Yang Heel Vessel)

Location: In a depression, directly below the tip of the lateral malleolus, in the articular cavity between the talus and calcaneus.

Depth of needling: 3 to 5 mm, perpendicularly.

Indication: Tension headache, psychovegetative dysregulation, peroneal neuralgia and paresis, dysfunction of the lower ankle joint (pronation, supination). Proven combination: SI 3 + B 62 for tension headache.
H. Schmidt: Pain in the inner corner of the eye.

Action in TCM: Removes obstruction from the meridian and collateral vessels, relaxes tendons and muscles, clears and calms the Mind (Shen), expels exterior pathogenic factors, opens the Yang Qiao Mai (Yang Heel Vessel).

○ B 67 "Zhi Yin"
   "Reaching Yin" ("Reaching Inside")
   Tonification Point

Location: Lateral corner of the nail of the fifth toe.

Depth of needling: 1 to 2 mm, perpendicularly; let it bleed if necessary.

Indication: Cephalalgia, urinary retention, uterine inertia; facilitating labor, correcting fetal malposition (moxa).
Caution! Needling during pregnancy is contraindicated.

Action in TCM: Removes obstructions from the meridian and collateral vessels, eliminates Wind, invigorates Blood, clears the eyes and the Mind (Shen).

Major Points of the Kidney Meridian

K 3: Source Point (Yuan Point).
K 6: Opening Point of the extraordinary meridian, Yin Qiao Mai (Yin Heel Vessel).
K 7: Tonification point.
K 27: Local point.

Points Associated with the Kidney Meridian

GB 25: Front Collecting Point (Mu Point) of the Kidney
B 23: Back Transporting Point (Back Shu Point) of the Kidney

Coupling Relationships of the Kidney Meridian

Top-to-bottom coupling:
Heart–Kidney

Yin-Yang coupling:
Kidney–Bladder

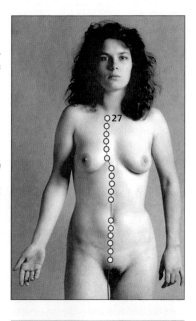

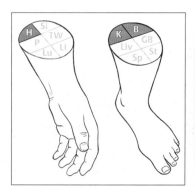

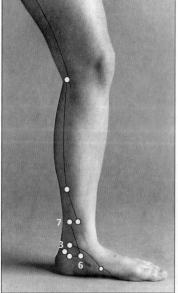

○ K 3 "Tai Xi"
"Greater Stream" ("Big Stream")
Source Point (Yuan Point)

Location: In the middle of the line connecting the greatest prominence of the medial malleolus with the Achilles tendon.

Depth of needling: 0.5 to 1 Cun, perpendicularly.

Indication: A prominent point for strengthening renal function and circulation; psychovegetative exhaustion, impotence, enuresis, painful menstruation, disorders of the urogenital tract, pain in the Achilles tendon, affections of the ankle joint.

Action in TCM: Supports Essence (Jing), bone and marrow, subdues Fire and cools Empty Heat (in case of Yin Deficiency), regulates the uterus, stabilizes emotions and the Mind (Shen).

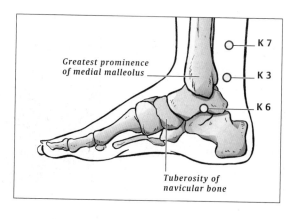

Greatest prominence of medial malleolus

K 7

K 3

K 6

Tuberosity of navicular bone

○ K 6 "Zhao Hai"
"Shining Sea" ("Shine on Sea")
Opening Point of the Extraordinary
Meridian, Yin Qiao Mai (Yin Heel
Vessel)

Location: 0.5 Cun caudal to the medial malleolus, in the region of the articular cavity between the talus and calcaneus, in the region of the sustentaculum tali. Point K 6 lies at the same level as Point B 62.

! The tibiocalcaneal part of the deltoid ligament expands between the medial malleolus and sustentaculum tali of the calcaneus. This ligament is important for stabilizing the inner malleolus. Many proprioceptors are found here in the vicinity of the lower ankle joint. The importance of the ankle joint functions for the entirety of harmonic human motions is also known to chiropractic.
Point K 6 is the Opening Point for the extraordinary meridian, Yin Qiao Mai. The translation of Qiao is "heel" (of the dancing girl), "mobility." Both Yin Qiao Mai and Yang Qiao Mai balance the Yang-Yin muscle tonus, regulate mobility of the joints, and affect the Bi syndrome (rheumatic symptoms).

Depth of needling: 0.3 to 0.5 Cun, perpendicularly.

Indication: Disorders of the urogenital tract; has a regulating activity on hormonal disorders, migraine, insomnia, night sweat, itching of the external genitals, general symptoms of chronic dryness (especially of the eyes), dry mucosa in the throat area, dry skin, dysfunction of the upper and lower ankle joints.
J. Bischko: A major point for emotional tonification.

Action in TCM: A prominent point for strengthening Kidney Yin and for general buildup of Yin; nourishes body fluids and moistens Dryness, supports the eyes and the throat, regulates the uterus, cools Heat and calms the Mind (Shen).

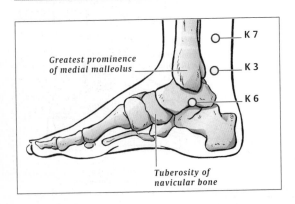

Greatest prominence of medial malleolus

K 7

K 3

K 6

Tuberosity of navicular bone

○ **K 7 "Fu Liu"**
   "Returning Current"
   ("Continuing Stream")
   Tonification Point

Location: 2 Cun above Point K 3, at the anterior margin of the Achilles tendon.

Depth of needling: 0.5 to 1 Cun, perpendicularly.

Indication: Important point for disorders of the urogenital tract, chronic lumbago and gonalgia, lack of motivation, depression, emotional and physical exhaustion, morning diarrhea.

Action in TCM: A prominent point for strengthening Kidney Yang and for general buildup of Yang (tonifies and stabilizes Yang), nourishes Yin, regulates Kidney Qi.

○ **K 27 "Shu Fu"**
   "Transport Point Mansion"
   ("Shu Mansion")

Location: Right under the clavicle, 2 Cun lateral to the median line in close proximity to the sternoclavicular joint.

Depth of needling: 2 to 4 mm, perpendicularly.
Caution! Deep needling carries the risk of pneumothorax.

Indication: Important point for treating asthma and pain in the chest.

Action in TCM: Subdues the rebellious Qi, regulates Lung Qi, tonifies Spleen and harmonizes Stomach, alleviates cough, supports Kidney in receiving Qi.

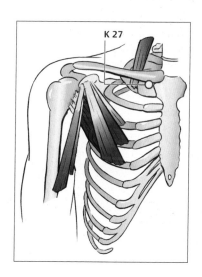

Major Points of the Pericardium Meridian

P 3: Local point.
P 6: Connecting Point (Luo Point). Opening Point of the extraordinary meridian, Yin Wei Mai (Yin Linking Vessel).
P 7: Source Point (Yuan Point).

Points Associated with the Pericardium Meridian

CV 17: Front Collecting Point (Mu Point) of the Pericardium
B 14: Back Transporting Point (Back Shu Point) of the Pericardium

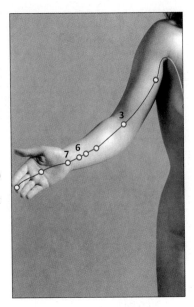

Coupling Relationships of the Pericardium Meridian

Top-to-bottom coupling:
Pericardium–Liver

Yin-Yang coupling:
Pericardium–Triple Warmer

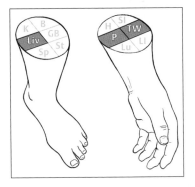

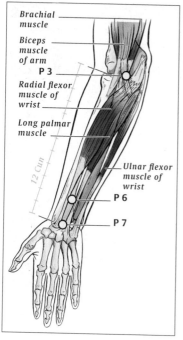

Brachial muscle

Biceps muscle of arm

P 3

Radial flexor muscle of wrist

Long palmar muscle

12 Cun

Ulnar flexor muscle of wrist

P 6

P 7

◎ **P 3 "Qu Ze"**
"Marsh on Bend" ("Crooked Marsh")

Location: Ulnar to the biceps tendon, in the crease of the elbow.

Depth of needling: 0.5 to 1 Cun, perpendicularly.

Indication: Epicondylopathy, angina pectoris, tachycardia, restlessness and panic attacks, fever and skin rashes, hypermenorrhea.

Action in TCM: Clears Heat and toxic Heat, cools Blood, circulates Blood and removes stagnation, calms Stomach, opens the orifices of the Heart, calms the Mind (Shen).

○ P 6 "Nei Guan"
"Inner Gate" ("Inner Pass")
Connecting Point (Luo Point)
Opening Point of the Extraordinary
Meridian, Yin Wei Mai (Yin Linking
Vessel)

Location: 2 Cun proximal to the crease of the wrist, between the tendons of the long palmar muscle and the radial flexor muscle of the wrist.
As described for localizing Point H 7, one should use the wrist crease that lies between the radius and ulna and the proximal carpal bones. The proximal carpal bones are marked by the pisiform bone; the crease in question is located proximal to the pisiform bone.

!
● For precise localization of the point, it is recommended to use the method of "dynamic palpation" which is described under Point TW 5. By palmar shifting of the skin fold between the radial flexor muscle of wrist and long palmar muscle in proximal direction, a distinct thickening of the fold is formed which becomes arrested at Point P 6. Point P 6 lies opposite to Point TW 5.

Depth of needling: 0.5 Cun, perpendicularly.

Indication: A point of overriding importance, prominent acupuncture point in case of pain and disorders in the thoracic and epigastric regions; has a strong emotionally harmonizing effect, especially in states of anxiety and agitation, functional heart problems, nausea, vomiting, singultus.

Action in TCM: Regulates the circulation of Qi, alleviates pain, opens the chest, regulates and clears the Middle Warmer, stimulates the descending of rebellious Stomach Qi, cools Heat, regulates Liver Qi and Blood, calms Heart and Mind (Shen).

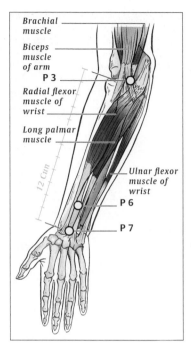

Brachial muscle
Biceps muscle of arm
P 3
Radial flexor muscle of wrist
Long palmar muscle
12 Cun
Ulnar flexor muscle of wrist
P 6
P 7

○ **P 7 "Da Ling"**
"Great Hill" ("Big Mound")
Source Point (Yuan Point)
Sedation Point

Location: In the middle of the wrist crease between the tendons of the long palmar muscle and the radial flexor muscle of wrist.
For help in localizing the wrist crease, see Point H 7.

Depth of needling: 0.3 to 0.5 Cun, perpendicularly.

Indication: Affections in the region of the wrist, enthesopathy in the region of the lower arm, functional heart problems, emotional states of agitation and anxiety. *J. Bischko:* Strong analgetic effect in the case of herpes zoster, writer's cramp.

Action in TCM: Calms Heart and Mind (Shen), cools Heat, Blood, Heart Heat, and Fire, removes stagnation.

Major Points of the Triple Warmer Meridian (San Jiao Meridian)*

TW 3: Tonification point.
TW 4: Source Point (Yuan Point).
TW 5: Connecting Point (Luo Point). Opening Point of the extraordinary meridian, Yang Wei Mai (Yang Linking Vessel).
TW 14: Local point.
TW 15: Local point.
TW 17: Local point.
TW 21: Local point.

Points Associated with the Triple Warmer Meridian

CV 5: Front Collecting Point (Mu Point) of the Triple Warmer.
B 22: Back Transporting Point (Back Shu Point) of the Triple Warmer.
B 39: Lower Sea Point (Lower He Point) of the Triple Warmer.

* Also known as Triple Burner (TB), Triple Energizer (TE, 3E), Triple Heater (TH).

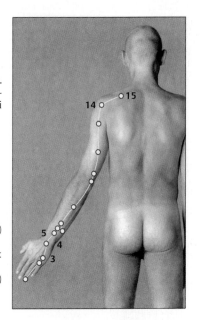

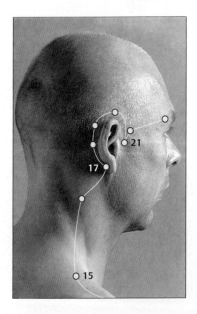

Coupling Relationships of the Triple Warmer Meridian

Top-to-bottom coupling:
Triple Warmer–Gall Bladder

Yin-Yang coupling:
Triple Warmer–Pericardium

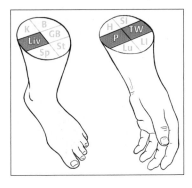

◉ TW 3 "Zhong Zhu"
"Middle Islet"
Tonification Point

Location: In a depression on the back of the hand between metacarpal bones IV and V, close to their body–head transition.

Depth of needling: 0.5 to 1 Cun, obliquely in proximal direction.

Indication: Important point for disorders of the ear, tinnitus, hearing difficulty, vertigo, cephalalgia, pain and paresis in the upper extremity.

Action in TCM: Opens the ear and promotes hearing, eliminates Heat and Wind Heat, expels Wind, removes obstructions from the meridian, clears head and eyes.

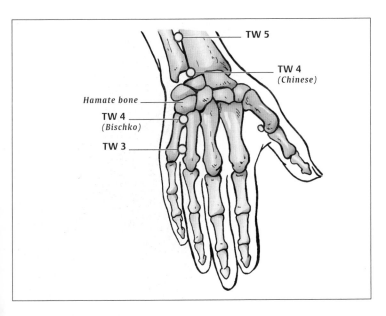

○ TW 4 "Yang Chi"
   "Yang Pond" ("Active Pond")
   Source Point (Yuan Point)

Location (Chinese): Slightly ulnar to the middle of the dorsal wrist crease (articular cavity between radius/ulna and proximal carpal bones), ulnar to the tendon of the extensor muscle of fingers, radial to the tendon of the extensor muscle of little finger.

> ! The tendon of the extensor muscle of fingers is best found by keyboard-playing exercises with the three long fingers. The dorsal wrist crease often becomes visible only upon dorsal flexion of the hand. If it is still indistinct even then, orientation takes place between the styloid processes of radius and ulna on a line running slightly convex in proximal direction.

According to *J. Bischko,* Point TW 4 is localized further distal, i.e., at the level of the articular cavity between metacarpal bones IV/V and the hamate bone. This point is often much more sensitive to pressure than the point localized according to the Chinese method. When in doubt, the decision is made by palpating for pressure sensitivity.

Depth of needling: Approx. 0.3 Cun, perpendicularly.

Indication: Wrist affections, pain and paresis in the upper extremity.
H. Schmidt: Moxibustion of Point TW 4 on the left hand has a general stimulating effect, especially on the organs of the lower abdomen.
J. Bischko: Master Point for vasomotor headache.

Action in TCM: Eliminates Wind Heat, relaxes tendons, removes obstructions from the meridian, benefits Original Qi (Yuan Qi).

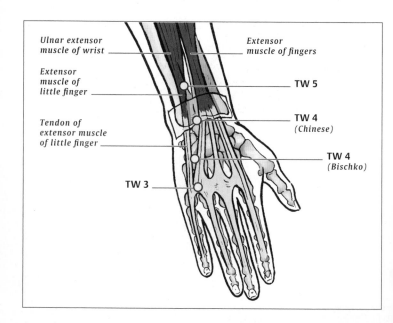

Ulnar extensor muscle of wrist

Extensor muscle of little finger

Tendon of extensor muscle of little finger

Extensor muscle of fingers

TW 5

TW 4 (Chinese)

TW 4 (Bischko)

TW 3

○ TW 5 "Wai Guan"
  "Outer Gate" ("Outer Pass")
  Connecting Point (Luo Point)
  Opening Point of the Extraordinary
  Meridian, Yang Wei Mai
  (Yang Linking Vessel)

Location: 2 Cun proximal to Point TW 4 between the radius and ulna (slightly ulnar to the middle of the dorsal wrist crease, see Point TW 4), on a line connecting Point TW 4 with the tip of the olecranon.

Advice: With the lower arm in supination (as shown in dorsal view in the fig. on p. 68), the connecting line lies roughly in the middle of the extensor muscle side of the lower arm. However, the lower arms are normally in pronation when the patient lies on his/her back. The connection line then runs clearly ulnar to the midline toward the olecranon. In this position of the arm, the line between Point TW 4 and the head of radius is used for orientation. Point TW 5 lies directly ulnar to this line.

!
● Point TW 5 can be found faster by dynamic palpation. For this purpose, the examiner's index finger slides from the dorsal wrist crease in proximal direction between the radius and ulna. At Point TW 5, the finger becomes arrested by the increasing thickening of the skin fold. Point TW 5 lies roughly oppositePoint P 6.

Depth of needling: 0.5 to 1 Cun, perpendicularly or in oblique proximal direction.

Indication: Cephalalgia, cervical syndrome, tinnitus, wrist affections, hearing difficulty; a major point for sensitivity to changes in the weather, pain and paresis in the upper extremity, feverish colds, skin eczema.
J. Bischko: Master Point for rheumatic complaints.

Action in TCM: A prominent point for removing the exterior pathogenic factors, especially Wind Heat, relieves the Exterior of the body, cools Heat and removes toxins, removes obstructions from the meridian, subdues ascending Liver Yang.

TW 14 "Jian Liao"
"Shoulder Crevice"

Location: In the posterior shoulder depression which forms when the arm is abducted by 90°, slightly caudal to the dorsal pole of the acromion.

> **!**
> ● Point TW 14 lies where the acromial part and the spinal part of the deltoid muscle come together. In muscular persons, the different components of the deltoid muscle (clavicular, acromial, and spinal parts) are prominent and the muscle grooves are easy to follow. Point TW 14 lies at the cranial end of the posterior groove, caudal to the dorsal pole of the acromion. The dorsal pole of the acromion can be found by following the course of the easily palpable scapular spine in lateral direction.

Depth of needling: 0.5 to 1.5 Cun, perpendicularly or in oblique distal direction.

Indication: Pain in the shoulder region; important local point.

Action in TCM: Eliminates exterior pathogenic factors such as Wind, Dampness, and Cold, removes obstructions from the meridian.

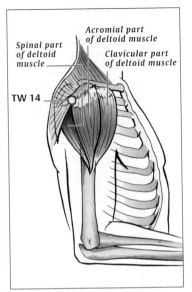

Spinal part of deltoid muscle

Acromial part of deltoid muscle

Clavicular part of deltoid muscle

TW 14

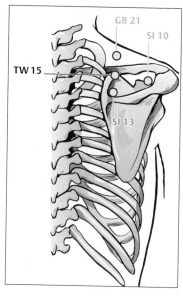

○ **TW 15 "Tian Liao"**
"Heavenly Crevice"
("Celestial Crevice")

Location: 1 Cun caudal to Point GB 21, in the middle between Points GB 21 and SI 13, on the superior angle of scapula.

> **!** Point GB 21 is localized in the middle between the lower edge of the spinous process of C7 and the acromion. (For help in localizing vertebra C7, see Point GB 21, p. 80.) Point SI 13 is localized in the middle of the lower edge of the spinous process of T2 and Point SI 10, in elongation of the dorsal fold of the arm pit, right above the scapula spine.

Depth of needling: 0.5 to 0.8 Cun, perpendicularly.
Caution! Risk of pneumothorax.

Indication: Cephalalgia, cervical syndrome, torticollis, sensitivity to changes in the weather.
B. Bischko: Master Point for the arms.

Action in TCM: Expels exterior pathogenic factors, such as Wind, Dampness, and Cold, removes obstructions from the meridian.

○ TW 17 "Yi Feng"
"Wind Screen" ("Shielding Wind")

Location: Behind the ear lobe, between the mandible and mastoid process.
Advice: Point TW 17 lies close to the facial nerve which exits from the stylomastoid foramen. There is the risk of puncturing the nerve when needling deeply.

Depth of needling: 0.5 to 1.5 Cun, perpendicularly or obliquely toward the front.

> ! ● The tip of the needle becomes positioned close to the transverse process of the atlas, which usually can be easily palpated between the mandible and mastoid process. This explains why the point has an effect on the upper head joints (see Indication).

Indication: Tinnitus, hearing difficulty, cephalalgia, trigeminal neuralgia, facial neuralgia, facial paresis, spasmolysis.
The upper head joints (atlanto-occipital joints) have an effect on the overall tonus of the body and play an important role as peripheral organ of balance.

Action in TCM: Expels Wind, removes obstructions from the meridian, cools Heat, promotes vision and hearing, relieves the senses.

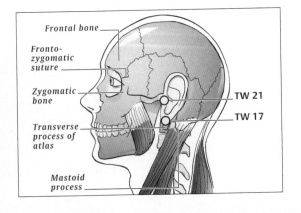

Frontal bone

Fronto-zygomatic suture

Zygomatic bone

Transverse process of atlas

Mastoid process

TW 21

TW 17

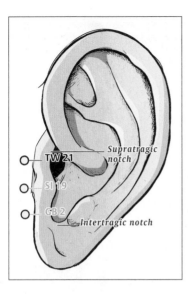

○ TW 21 "Er Men"
"Ear Door" ("Ear Gate")

Location: At the level of the supratragic notch above Point SI 19 immediately behind the upper dorsal portion of the condylar process of mandible.

❗ The needle is inserted with the mouth slightly opened. This way, the temporomandibular joint moves slightly in ventral direction so that there is no risk of injuring it (depth of needling, approx. 0.5 Cun). The mouth is closed after inserting the needle. Subcutaneous needling in the direction of Points SI 19 and GB 2 is also possible. By moving the needle forward more or less deeply, these points are also influenced and the effect of Point TW 21 is increased (same indications for SI 19 and GB 2 as for TW 21).

Advice: Point TW 21 lies in close proximity to the superficial temporal artery; puncture of this vessel can be avoided by palpating its pulse prior to needling.

Depth of needling: 0.5 Cun, perpendicularly or subcutaneously in caudal direction.

Indication: Disorders of the ear, gnathological disorders, toothache, cephalalgia.

Action in TCM: Opens the ear, promotes hearing, removes obstructions from the meridian, cools Heat.

Major Points of the Gall Bladder Meridian

GB 2: Local point.
GB 8: Local point.
GB 14: Local point.
GB 20: Point with broad regulatory effect on Wind Diseases.
GB 21: Local point.
GB 30: Local point.
GB 34: Lower Sea Point (Lower He Point) of the Gall Bladder. Master Point of the muscles and tendons.
GB 39: Master Point of the marrow.
GB 41: Opening Point of the extraordinary meridian, Dai Mai (Girdle Vessel).

Points Associated with the Gall Bladder Meridian

GB 24: Front Collecting Point (Mu Point) of the Gall Bladder.
B 19: Back Transporting Point (Back Shu Point) of the Gall Bladder.
GB 34: Lower Sea Point (Lower He Point) of the Gall Bladder.

Coupling Relationships of the Gall Bladder Meridian
Top-to-bottom coupling:

Triple Warmer–Gall Bladder

Yin-Yang coupling:
Gall Bladder–Liver

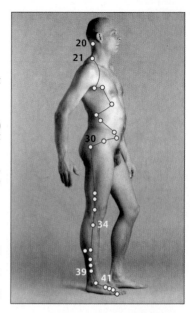

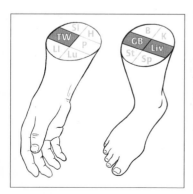

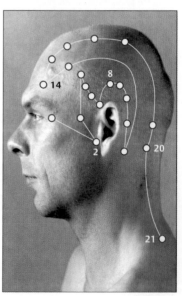

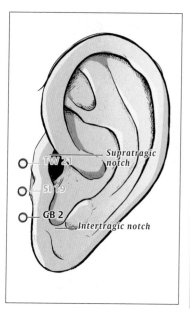

Supratragic notch

TW 21

SI 19

GB 2

Intertragic notch

○ **GB 2 "Ting Hui"**
"Hearing Convergence"
("Listening Convergence")

Location: In front of the intertragic notch, directly below Point SI 19 (depression in front of the tragus when the mouth is slightly opened), in front of the posterior edge of the condylar process of mandible.

! The needle is inserted with the mouth slightly opened so that the temporomandibular joint moves slightly in ventral direction. This way, there is no risk of injuring the joint (depth of needling, approx. 0.5 Cun). The mouth is closed after inserting the needle.
In case of ear disorders, the space Points TW 21, SI 19, and GB 2 can all be reached with the same needle. For this purpose, the needle is pushed subcutaneously in caudal direction until Point GB 2 is reached.

Advice: Point GB 2 lies close to the superficial temporal artery; puncture of this vessel can be avoided by palpating its pulse prior to needling.

Depth of needling: 0.5 to 1 Cun, perpendicularly (see note above).

Indication: Gnathological problems, disorders of the ear, migraine, tinnitus, toothache.

Action in TCM: Expels exterior Wind, removes obstructions from the meridian, opens the ears and supports hearing.

○ **GB 8 "Shuai Gu"**
"Leading the Valley"
("Following the Valley")

Location: 1.5 Cun above the highest point of the auricula.

Depth of needling: 0.3 to 0.5 Cun, obliquely in the direction of the site of pain.

Indication: Parietal and temporal cephalalgia.
J. Bischko: Needling of Point GB 8 on both sides of the head and of Point GV 20 (Du Mai 20) causes a horizontal flow through the head, while a vertical flow is promoted by needling the following points: PdM (Point de Merveille; also called Yin Tang, EX-HN 3), GV 16, and GV 20.

Action in TCM: Opens the ear and supports hearing, removes obstructions from the meridian, expels exterior Wind.

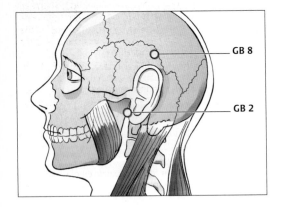

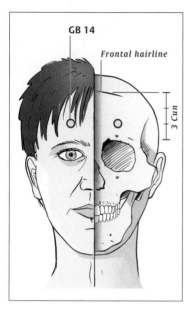

GB 14

Frontal hairline

3 Cun

GB 14 "Yang Bai" "Yang White"

Location: 1 Cun above the middle of the eyebrow, right above the pupil when looking straight ahead. The total distance between mid eyebrow and frontal hairline is 3 Cun; hence, Point GB 14 lies at the end of the first third of this distance.

> **!** In case of baldness, the border of the original hairline can be demonstrated by frowning.

Depth of needling: 0.3 to 0.5 Cun, subcutaneously toward the site of pain (site of disturbed function).

Indication: Cephalalgia, trigeminal neuralgia, sinusitis, disturbed vision. Point GB 14 is particularly sensitive to pressure in case of disorders in the gall bladder region (prominent trigger point). The combination of GB 14 and GB 20 improves the flow through the head in the sense of front–back coupling (compare with Point GB 8).
J. Bischko: Test point for disorders of the gall bladder.

Action in TCM: Purges exterior and interior Wind and Wind Heat, cools Heat, opens the eyes and promotes vision.

○ **GB 20 "Feng Chi"**
"Wind Pond"

Location: In a depression between the insertions of sternocleidomastoid muscle and trapezius muscle at the lower edge of the occiput.
The needle is inserted at the level between occiput and atlas (upper head joints) in the region of the transverse process of atlas; it passes through the splenius capitis muscle, then through the semispinalis capitis muscle and becomes positioned close to the obliquus capitis superior and inferior muscles.

Depth of needling: Approximately 1 Cun in the direction of the contralateral eye socket or the contralateral upper incisor region (depending on head position).

! The vertebral artery is located at a considerable depth of 4 cm (often more). Point GB 20 is usually treated by deep needling, as the Qi sensation can often be induced only this way. In slim patients, however, the depth of needling should not exceed 2 cm.

Indication: All diseases the symptoms of which resemble Wind (i.e., those appearing suddenly) vary in localization and intensity (e.g., cervical syndrome, facial paresis, tinnitus, conjunctivitis, allergies, influenza or flu-like infections).
J. Bischko: Master Point for Wind diseases, Master Point of the sympathetic nervous system, used in all cases of disease where we find an excessive reaction of the sympathetic nervous system (hypertension,

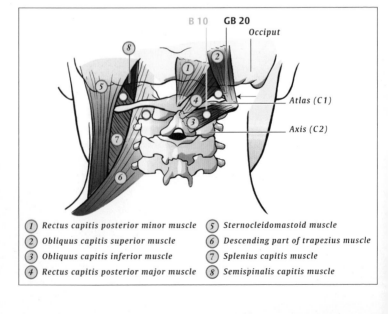

B 10   **GB 20**
Occiput

Atlas (C1)

Axis (C2)

① *Rectus capitis posterior minor muscle*
② *Obliquus capitis superior muscle*
③ *Obliquus capitis inferior muscle*
④ *Rectus capitis posterior major muscle*
⑤ *Sternocleidomastoid muscle*
⑥ *Descending part of trapezius muscle*
⑦ *Splenius capitis muscle*
⑧ *Semispinalis capitis muscle*

tinnitus, vertigo, vegetative dysregula-tion, influenza or other infections, mi-graine), tension in the body (affecting the overall tonus of the body, see below) such as migraine, tension headache, premen-strual syndrome, dysmenorrhea, and, fi-nally, vertigo and imbalance (regulation of balance, see below).

The point is often needled in combina-tion with Point B 10, the Master Point of the parasympathetic nervous system (*J. Bischko*).

The point's localization explains the posi-tive effect of GB 20 on tension in the neck muscles of the head joint region as well as blockage of the head joints. Via re-flexes, afferent nerves from the head joint region have an effect on:

▶ autonomic regulation (there are neural connections to autonomic centers);
▶ overall tonus of the body (by affecting the gamma system which controls the overall tonus of the body);
▶ regulation of balance (the upper cervi-cal spine, in particular, is an important organ of balance).

Many of the indications listed can be ex-plained by means of points in the head joint region. Also the term "Master Point of the sympathetic nervous system" ac-cording to *J. Bischko* has a conventional medical explanation (see also Point B 10).

Action in TCM: A prominent point for eliminating exterior and interior Wind; calms Liver Yang, cools Liver Fire and Heat, relaxes muscles and tendons, re-moves obstructions from the meridian, clears head and eyes, relieves the senses, harmonizes Qi and Blood, promotes hear-ing and vision.

○ GB 21 "Jian Jing"
"Shoulder Well"

Location: In the middle of the line connecting the acromion with the spinous process of C7, on the dorsal vertical extension of the mamillary line.

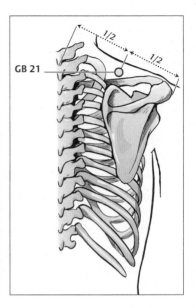

!
● How to localize C7: The spinous process of C7 is the first of the cervical spine which does not slide ventrally upon retroflexion of the head. During palpation it is recommended to search first for the most prominent spinous process (probably C7) while in anteflexion and to mark it with the tip of the finger. Upon retroflexion, the finger remains in place, provided the process is that of C7; if the finger moves in ventral direction, it is that of C6. Examination with two fingers is also possible: one finger is placed on the presumed C6 process, the other one on the C7 process. Upon retroflexion, one can feel the ventral gliding of the upper process and the two spinous processes approaching each other.

Depth of needling: 0.5 to 1 Cun, perpendicularly to the skin surface, or by using the dry-needling method.

Indication: Pain in shoulder and neck, headache, facilitation of child birth, retained placenta, difficult lactation, mastitis.
Point GB 21 corresponds to a common trigger point.

Action in TCM: Relaxes the tendons, removes obstructions from the meridian, descends Qi, promotes uterine contraction and lactation.

○ **GB 30 "Huan Tiao"**
"Jumping Circle" ("Circular Jump")

Location: Lateral side of the hip, on the connecting line between the greater trochanter and sacral hiatus, between the outer and middle third of the line. In China, this point is always needled with the patient in lateral position. Hip and knee of the side to be treated are flexed, while the lower leg is extended.

Depth of needling: 1.5 to 3 Cun, perpendicularly.

Indication: Lumbago, lumbago–sciatica syndrome; important sciatica point; neuralgia-like symptoms and paresis of the lower extremity, coxalgia.

Action in TCM: Removes obstructions from the meridian, expels Wind, Cold, and Dampness from the meridian, strengthens the lower back and the hip.

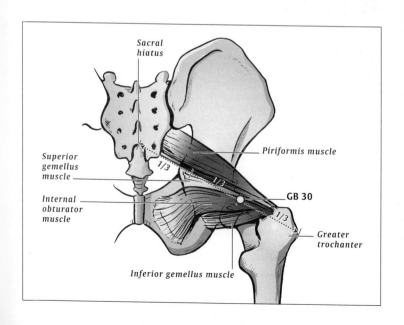

○ GB 34 "Yang Ling Quan"
"Yang Hill Spring"
("Yang Mound Spring")
Lower Sea Point (Lower He Point) of
the Gall Bladder
Master Point of the Muscles and
Tendons

Location: In the depression in front of and below the head of fibula.

! To find this point, it is recommended to search first for the head of fibula in the region where the trouser seam would be. The head of fibula is then gripped between index and middle fingers with both fingers sliding caudally. Point GB 34 is found under the index finger, directly below and in front of the head of fibula. Needling takes place in the direction of the interosseous membrane, i.e., between tibia and fibula. When the knee is flexed, searching for the head of fibula is achieved by following the course of the clearly palpable tendon of the biceps muscle of thigh, which runs toward the head of fibula.

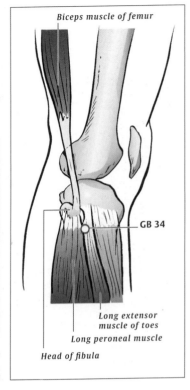

Biceps muscle of femur

GB 34

Long extensor
muscle of toes
Long peroneal muscle
Head of fibula

Advice: Needling Point GB 34 may irritate deep fibers of the deep fibular nerve. Puncture of the common fibular nerve is also possible in case it is located high.

Depth of needling: 1 to 2 Cun, obliquely toward the interosseous membrane between the tibia and fibula.

Indication: Myalgia, gonalgia, coxalgia, pain and paresis in the lower extremity, tinnitus, cephalalgia, hypertension.

Action in TCM: Most important point for promoting the free flow of Liver Qi, relaxes the tendons, regulates Liver and Gall Bladder, calms Liver Yang and Liver Wind, removes Damp Heat, eliminates Moisture and Phlegm, removes obstructions from the meridian.

○ **GB 39 "Xuan Zhong"**
"Hanging Bell" ("Suspended Bell")
Meridians of the Foot
Master Point of the Marrow

Location: 3 Cun above the highest prominence of the lateral malleolus, at the anterior edge of the fibula. The Chinese literature (Chinese Acupuncture and Moxibustion) sometimes localizes Point GB 39 at the posterior edge of the fibula. The decision is made by palpating for pressure sensitivity.

Depth of needling: 0.5 to 2 Cun, perpendicularly.

Indication: Acute torticollis, cephalalgia (Fullness), cervical syndrome.

Action in TCM: Benefits Essence (Jing), nourishes the marrow, calms Liver Wind, expels Heat, removes Damp Heat.

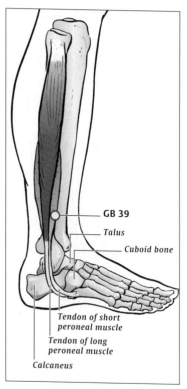

GB 39

Talus

Cuboid bone

Tendon of short
peroneal muscle

Tendon of long
peroneal muscle

Calcaneus

○ **GB 41 "Zu Lin Qi"**
"Falling Tears" ("Above Tears")
Opening Point of the Extraordinary
Meridian, Dai Mai (Girdle Vessel)

Location: At the body–base transition of metatarsal bones IV and V, lateral to the tendon of the long extensor muscle of toes running toward the little toe.

! Finding the base of metatarsal bone V is most accurately achieved from the lateral edge of the foot. Starting from the clearly palpable base, palpation is performed distal to the body–base transition of metatarsal bone V. From here, palpation continues in medial direction along the extended line between the fourth and fifth toes. If involved, Point GB 41 is clearly pressure sensitive.

Depth of needling: 0.3 to 0.5 Cun, perpendicularly.

Indication: Migraine, joint disorders, pain in the lateral regions of head, thorax, and abdomen, mastitis, lumbago–sciatica syndrome.

Action in TCM: Promotes the smooth flow of Liver Qi, calms Liver Yang and Liver Wind, purges Heat, removes Damp Heat from the Lower Warmer, regulates the Dai Mai (Girdle Vessel), strengthens vision and hearing.

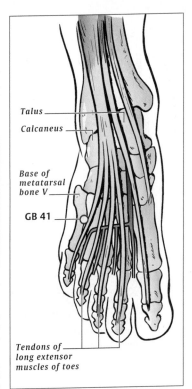

Talus

Calcaneus

Base of metatarsal bone V

GB 41

Tendons of long extensor muscles of toes

Major Points of the Liver Meridian

Liv 2: Sedation point.
Liv 3: Source Point (Yuan Point).
Liv 13: Front Collecting Point (Mu Point) of the Spleen. Master Point of the Zang organs.
Liv 14: Front Collecting Point (Mu Point) of the Liver.

Points Associated with the Liver Meridian

Liv 14: Front Collecting Point (Mu Point) of the Liver.
B 18: Back Transporting Point (Back Shu Point) of the Liver.

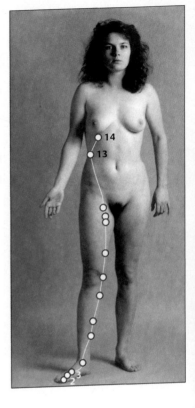

Coupling Relationships of the Liver Meridian

Top-to-bottom coupling:
Pericardium–Liver

Yin-Yang coupling:
Liver–Gall Bladder

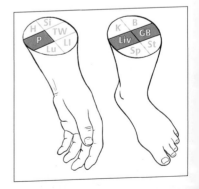

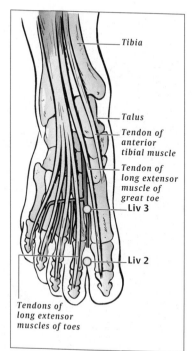

Tibia

Talus

Tendon of anterior tibial muscle

Tendon of long extensor muscle of great toe

Liv 3

Liv 2

Tendons of long extensor muscles of toes

○ **Liv 2 "Xing Jian"**
"Temporary In-between"
("Between Columns")
Sedation Point

Location: Proximal to the end of the interdigital fold between the first and second toes.

Depth of needling: 0.5 to 1 Cun, perpendicularly.

Indication: Spastic pain (especially in the gynecological region), cephalalgia, glaucoma, pain and paresis in the lower extremity, thoracodynia, vertigo, tinnitus, insomnia.

Action in TCM: Important point in acute cases of Liver Fullness (Liver Fire, ascending Liver Yang); cools Heat and purges Fire, regulates Liver Qi, cools Blood Heat, subdues interior Wind, removes Damp Heat from the Lower Warmer.

○ **Liv 3 "Tai Chong"**
"Bigger Rushing" ("Great Rush")
Source Point (Yuan Point)

Location: In the proximal corner between metatarsal bones I and II where body and base regions of both bones come closer.

Depth of needling: 0.5 to 1 Cun, perpendicularly, perhaps in slightly proximal direction.

Indication: Spasmolytic effect (often used in combination with Liv 2), cephalalgia, obstipation, diarrhea, liver and gall bladder problems, important distal point for the urogenital region, hypertension, vertigo, eye disorders.

Action in TCM: Cools Heat in Liver and Gall Bladder, regulates Liver Qi and stagnation of Blood, calms Liver Yang, expels Liver Wind, opens the eyes, calms the Mind (Shen), removes Damp Heat from the Lower Warmer.

○ **Liv 13 "Zhang Men"**
"Chapter Gate" ("Bright Door")
Front Collecting Point (Mu Point)
of the Spleen
Master Point of the Zang Organs

Location: At the free end of the eleventh rib, at the lateral side of abdomen.

Depth of needling: 0.5 Cun, obliquely.

Indication: Liver and gall bladder diseases, indigestion, metabolic disorders, vomiting.

Action in TCM: Tonifies Spleen, removes stagnation of Food, regulates the flow of Liver Qi, promotes circulation of Blood, removes stagnation of Blood.

○ **Liv 14 "Qi Men"**
"Cyclic Gate" ("Cycle Door")
Front Collecting Point (Mu Point)
of the Liver

Location: In the sixth intercostal space (ICS 6) below the mamilla on the mamillary line.

! How to localize the ICS: The transition of sternal manubrium–sternal body is clearly palpable. Lateral to it is the second rib, and below this is ICS 2.

Depth of needling: 0.5 Cun, obliquely along the course of the rib.

Indication: Liver disease, indigestion, intercostal neuralgia, vertigo.

Action in TCM: Promotes the smooth flow of Liver Qi, removes stagnation of Liver Qi and Blood, transforms Phlegm, cools Blood Heat, promotes lactation.

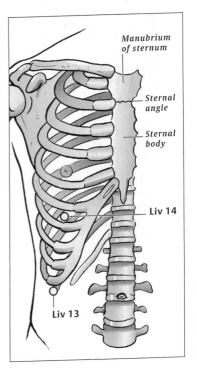

Manubrium of sternum

Sternal angle

Sternal body

Liv 14

Liv 13

Major Points of the Conception Vessel

CV 3: Front Collecting Point (Mu Point) of the Bladder.

CV 4: Front Collecting Point (Mu Point) of the Small Intestine.

CV 6: General tonification point.

CV 8: General tonification point.

CV 12: Front Collecting Point (Mu Point) of the Stomach. Master Point of the Fu organs. Front Collecting Point (Mu Point) of the Middle Warmer.

CV 17: Front Collecting Point (Mu Point) of the Pericardium. Master Point of the respiratory tract. Front Collecting Point (Mu Point) of the Upper Warmer.

CV 22: Local point.

CV 24: Local point.

Points Associated with the Conception Vessel

Lu 7: Opening Point of the Conception Vessel.

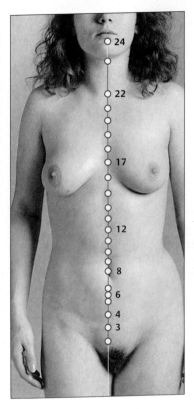

○ **CV 3 "Zhong Ji"**
"Middle Extremity"
("Middle Extreme")
Front Collecting Point (Mu Point) of the Bladder

Location: 1 Cun cranial to the middle of the upper edge of the symphysis.

> ● When using Cun as a measure in the abdominal region, it is very important to take the distance between the upper edge of the symphysis and the navel—5 Cun—as guidance. This is the only way of taking into account the differences in abdominal girth; it cannot be accomplished with the usual thumb–Cun measure.

Depth of needling: 1 to 1.5 Cun, perpendicularly.

Indication: Disorders of the urogenital tract, incontinence, disordered menstruation (such as dysmenorrhea, amenorrhea, irregular period), female infertility, vaginal discharge, postpartum hemorrhage, postpartum afterpains, pain and itching of the exterior genitals, impotence, premature ejaculation.

Action in TCM: Eliminates Damp Heat in the Lower Warmer, regulates the flow of Qi, expels Heat, regulates the uterus.

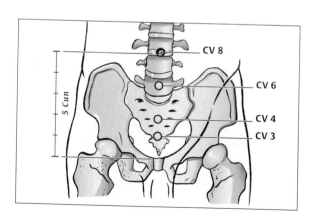

○ **CV 4 "Guan Yuan"**
  "Gate of the Original Qi"
  ("Energy Pass")
  **Front Collecting Point (Mu Point) of
  the Small Intestine**

Location: 2 Cun cranial to the middle of the upper edge of the symphysis (for accurate orientation, see Point CV 3).

Depth of needling: 1 to 1.5 Cun, perpendicularly.

Indication: A prominent point for treating urogenital and gynecological syndromes; important tonification point in case of emotional and physical exhaustion, abdominal complaints, persistent postpartum hemorrhage.
König/Wancura: CV 4 + Sp 6: Basic point combination for disorders of the urogenital tract.

> ❗ Point CV 4 represents the intersection of the interior branches of the Three Yin Meridians of the Foot. This explains the broad effect on gynecological syndromes and disorders of the urogenital tract, similar to the effect of Point Sp 6 (intersection of the exterior, point-carrying parts of the Three Yin Meridians of the Foot).

Action in TCM: Nourishes Blood and Yin, warms the uterus and the Lower Warmer, invigorates Kidney, Yang, and Original Qi (Yuan Qi), expels Dampness and Cold from the Lower Warmer.

○ **CV 6 "Qi Hai"**
  "Sea of Qi" ("Energy Sea")

Location: 1.5 Cun below the navel (for accurate orientation, see Point CV 3).

Depth of needling: 1 to 1.5 Cun, perpendicularly.

Indication: Prominent tonification point in case of emotional and physical exhaustion, often used with moxa; exhaustion, circulatory dysregulation, impotence.

Action in TCM: Tonifies Qi and Yang, tonifies Original Qi (Yuan Qi), regulates and promotes circulation of Qi, warms and invigorates the Lower and Middle Warmer, removes stagnation of Qi, removes Dampness.

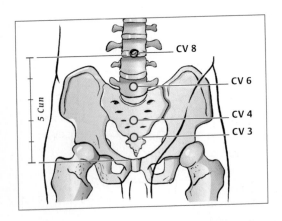

5 Cun

CV 8
CV 6
CV 4
CV 3

○ **CV 8 "Shen Que"**
 "Mind Palace" ("Navel")

Location: In the center of the navel.

> ❗ One possibility of providing energy in case of general states of exhaustion is to apply navel moxibustion with moxa, ginger, and salt (three Yang substances).

Indication: Positively no needling! It often makes sense to use moxibustion for general tonification.

Action in TCM: Tonifies Yang, Spleen, and Original Qi.

○ **CV 12 "Zhong Wan"**
 "Middle of Epigastrium" ("Center of Power")
 Front Collecting Point (Mu Point) of the Stomach
 Master Point of the Fu Organs
 Front Collecting Point (Mu Point) of the Middle Warmer

Location: In the middle of the line connecting the base of the xiphoid with the navel.

> ❗ As with the lower abdomen, it is important to take the distance between the base of the xiphoid (intersection of costal arches) and the navel—8 Cun—as guidance for points of the upper abdomen. This is the only way that differences in the abdominal girth can be taken into account.

Depth of needling: 1 to 1.5 Cun, perpendicularly.

Indication: A prominent point in all disorders of the gastrointestinal tract; gastritis, ulcers of stomach and duodenum, meteorism, gastrocardiac syndrome, nausea, vomiting, singultus, insomnia.

Action in TCM: Tonifies Stomach and Spleen, regulates Stomach Qi, stimulates the descending of rebellious Stomach Qi, transforms Dampness.

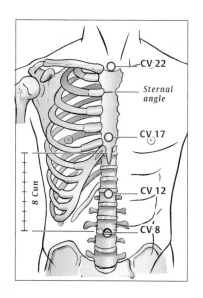

○ **CV 17 "Dan Zhong"**
"Middle of Chest"
("Sea of Tranquility")
Front Collecting Point (Mu Point)
of the Pericardium
Master Point of the Respiratory Tract
Front Collecting Point (Mu Point)
of the Upper Warmer

Location: On the median line at the level of the mamillae, in ICS 4.

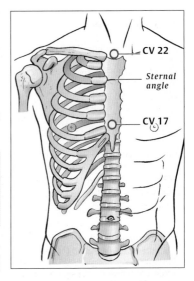

❗ ● The distance between the upper edge of the sternal manubrium and the base of the xiphoid measures 9 Cun. However, orientation usually takes place by determining the intercostal space.

Depth of needling: 0.3 to 0.5 Cun, subcutaneously in caudal direction toward the tip of the xiphoid process, or in lateral direction toward the mamilla.

❗ ● The osseous lamina in the region of Point CV 17 may be anatomically very thin (due to disturbed sternal ossification during embryonic development); foramina may even be present and hence the risk of intracardiac puncture.
A more or less prominent sternal foramen is found in 8–10% of the population; a thin osseous lamina or connective-tissue membrane may render the results of the palpation inconspicuous. The distance between the skin surface and the dorsal surface of the sternum measures only 12 to 22 mm. Cases of death have been reported. Hence, needling should be strictly tangential.
For palpation of ICS 4, it is recommended to search first for the clearly palpable transition of the sternal angle between sternal manubrium and sternal corpus. Lateral to it lies the second rib, caudal to it lies ICS 2.

Indication: A prominent point in case of acute and chronic breathing difficulties, bronchial asthma, bronchitis, dyspnea, thoracodynia, functional heart problems, sensation of tightness in the thorax.

Action in TCM: Regulates and promotes circulation of Qi in the Upper Warmer, tonifies the Gathering Qi of the chest (Zong Qi), opens the chest, removes viscous Phlegm, stimulates the descending of rebellious Lung Qi and Stomach Qi.

CV 22 "Tian Tu"
"Heaven Projection"
("Sky Prominence")

Location: In the middle of the jugular notch of the sternum, at the level of the attachment of the clavicle.

Method of needling: According to Chinese literature, Point CV 22 is needled deeply retrosternally in acute attacks of asthma.

Depth of needling: 0.5 to 1 Cun, retrosternally.

Indication: Bronchial asthma, singultus, globus sensation, hoarseness.
Caution! In the case of needling too deeply and in the case of infections, there is a risk of mediastinitis because of interconnecting spaces in the connective tissue.

Action in TCM: Stimulates the descending of rebellious Lung Qi, clears Heat and viscous Phlegm from the larynx and thorax, strengthens the voice, calms cough.

CV 24 "Cheng Jiang"
"Saliva Receiver" ("Receiving Saliva")

Location: The deepest site of the mandibular median line, in the middle of the mentolabial crease.

! If needling is carried out for the purpose of reducing an excessive pharyngeal reflex (e.g., during endoscopic examination, or while taking a cast), it is recommended to use a very short needle prior to the examination. If the needle is bent in the region of the handle, it may remain in place during examination.

Depth of needling: 0.2 to 0.3 Cun, perpendicularly.

Indication: Facial pain, toothache, facial paresis, trigeminal neuralgia, hypersalivation, facial spasm, reduction of an excessive pharyngeal reflex in the case of endoscopic examination as well as dental interventions (taking a cast).

Action in TCM: Expels exterior Wind, reduces facial swelling and pain.

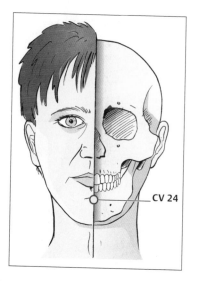

CV 24

Major Points of the Governor Vessel

GV 4: General tonification point.
GV 14: Crossing Point of all Yang Meridians.
GV 15: Local point.
GV 16: Local point.
GV 20: Local point with systemic effect.
GV 26: Local point, emergency point.

Point Associated with the Governor Vessel

SI 3: Opening Point of the Governor Vessel.

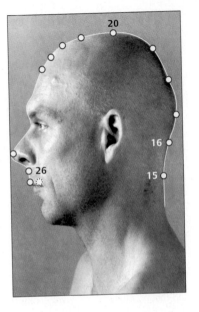

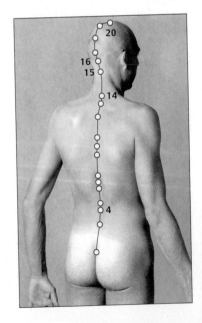

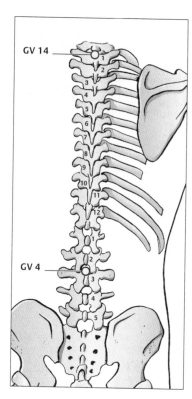

○ **GV 4 "Ming Men"**
"Gate of Life"

Location: Below the spinous process of L2.
Point GV 4 lies at the same level as Point B 23. An interior branch of the Kidney Meridian joins here; Point GV 4 therefore enhances the effect of Point B 23.

Depth of needling: 0.5 to 1 Cun, perpendicularly or, perhaps, in oblique caudal direction.

! ● The literature describes very rare cases of injuries to the spinal cord following extremely deep needling in cranial direction. Insertion of the needle in the described direction should therefore not exceed 1 Cun, or the needle should be guided perpendicularly or in slightly caudal direction.

Indication: A prominent point for tonifying Yang and especially Kidney Yang; lumbago, urogenital disorders, sexual dysfunction, tinnitus, cephalalgia.

! ● Point GV 4 as well as Point B 23 have a tonifying effect on dysfunctions of the kidney and bladder. They are indicated in patients with symptoms of Cold, Weakness, and Emptiness.
Needling or moxibustion of this "dorsal tonification line for lumbago" is recommended in case of concurrent lumbago. If appropriate (when sensitive to pressure), additional needling or moxibustion of Point B 52 (1.5 Cun lateral to Point B 23) is an option. Instead of needling Points B 23 and B 52 as described, moxa platelets or "hot spots" (self-warming, scent-neutral platelets) may be also used.

Action in TCM: Tonifies Kidney Yang and Original Qi (Yuan Qi), benefits Essence (Jing), warms the Gate of Life (Ming Men), strengthens the back, legs, and knees, expels Cold.

○ GV 14 "Da Zhui"
  "Big Vertebra"

Location: Below the spinous process of C7.

> ! How to find the spinous process of C7: In contrast to C6, C7 does not slide forward when reclining the head. Examination is performed by placing the middle and index fingers on the supposed spinous processes of C6 and C7. If the fingers are correctly positioned, they move toward each other when the head is reclined and the upper spinous process swerves in ventral direction.

Depth of needling: 0.5 to 1 Cun, perpendicularly.

Indication: Cephalalgia; the point has an immunomodulating effect; fever, paralysis, tinnitus.

J. Bischko: A Crossing Point with connections to the six Fu organs. (In combination with other points, this point is also called the "spider".)
Point GV 14 has an effect on all Yang Meridians; quick orientation in case of headache and neck pain takes place by palpating the major points of the "spider" around Point GV 14.

> ! Not all points of the "spider" are needled. Only those most sensitive to pressure are selected.

Action in TCM: Removes exterior pathogenic factors from the Yang Meridians, expels Wind Heat, relieves the Exterior of the body, circulates Blood, calms the Mind (Shen).

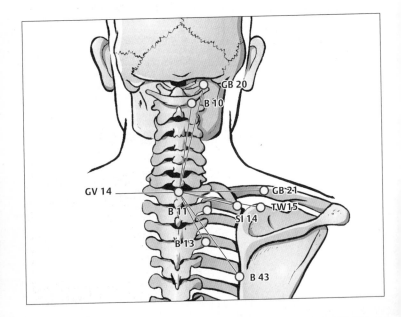

○ GV 15 "Ya Men"
"Gate of Dumbness" ("Dumb Gate")

Location: Above the spinous process of C2 at the same level as Point B 10, 0.5 Cun above the dorsal hairline.

Depth of needling: 0.5 Cun, in slightly caudal direction.

● When needling both Point GV 15 and Point GV 16: needling is carried out in slightly caudal direction with the head bent slightly forward. The tip of the needle should be positioned in the nuchal ligament. Do not stimulate. When needling Point GV 16 too deeply, there is a risk of penetrating into the cerebellomedullary cistern.

Indication: An important point for speech disorder, especially in children; aphasia, general speech disorders, epilepsy, apoplexy, cervical syndrom, stiffness of the neck, occipital pain.

Action in TCM: Stimulates speech, lightens up the senses, clears the Mind (Shen), purges Heat, suppresses interior Wind.

○ GV 16 "Feng Fu"
"Wind Palace" ("Windy Mansion")

Location: Below the exterior occipital protuberance at the same level as Point GB 20.

Depth of needling: 0.5 Cun, in slightly caudal direction (see Point GV 15).

● See Point GV 15.

Indication: Cephalalgia; promotes longitudinal flow through the head (in combination with Point EX-HN 1); tinnitus, confusion; a prominent point for exterior and interior Wind diseases; vertigo, rhinitis, sinusitis.

Action in TCM: When using the sedation method: expels exterior and interior Wind (apart from GB 20, the most important point for eliminating Wind), clears the Mind (Shen);
when using the tonification method: invigorates brain functions, benefits the Mind (Shen).

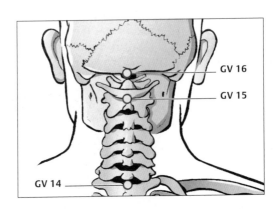

○ GV 20 "Bai Hui"
   "Hundred Meetings"
   ("Hundred Convergences")

Location: On the median line of the head, 5 Cun into the hair from the frontal hair line, on a line connecting the tips of both ears. In German-language literature, the ear axis (see fig.) is often pointed out as a guide for localizing the tip of the ear and the connecting line.

Depth of needling: 0.5 Cun, subcutaneously toward the front or the back.

Indication: An important sedation point; emotional harmonization; cephalalgia, insomnia, vertigo, symptoms of anxiety (apart from Points Ll 4 and St 36, one of the most often used points).

Action in TCM: Expels interior Wind, clears and calms the Mind (Shen), calms Liver Wind and Liver Yang, opens the sensory organs.

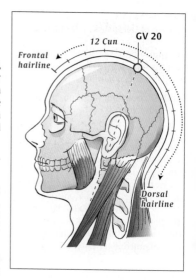

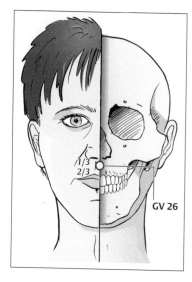

○ **GV 26 "Shui Gou"**
"Water Groove"
Also known as "Ren Zhong"
"Middle of Person"
("Middle of Man")

Location: In the philtrum on the frontal median line, between the nasal third and the remaining two-thirds of the connecting line between nose and upper lip margin.

Depth of needling: 0.5 Cun, obliquely in cranial direction.

Indication: Collapse, epileptic seizure, acute lumbago.

!
In emergency cases (when no needles are available), it is recommended to use firm acupressure with the thumb against the lower edge of the nose.

Action in TCM: Opens the senses, calms the Mind (Shen) and restores consciousness, cools Heat, suppresses Wind, supports the back.

In China there has been an official agreement since 1991 on 48 Extra Points. This agreement is supported by the WHO. The extrapoints are named after the respective region of the body, and their number varies from region to region.

English Names:	Number of Points:
EX-HN (Head–Neck)	15
EX-CA (Chest–Abdomen)	1
EX-B (Back)	9
EX-UE (Upper Extremity)	1
EX-LE (Lower Extremity)	12

Chinese name	English name	Chinese Acupuncture & Moxibustion
Shi Shen Cong	EX-HN 1	Extra 6
Yin Tang	EX-HN 3	Extra 2
Yu Yao	EX-HN 4	Extra 5
Tai Yang	EX-HN 5	Extra 1
Jing Bai Lao	EX-HN 15	Extra 16
Ding Chuan	EX-B 1	Extra 14
Hua Tuo Jia Ji	EX-B 2	Extra 15
Shi Qi Zhui	EX-B 8	Extra 18
Wai Lao Gong/Luo Zhen	EX-UE 8	Extra 28
Ba Xie	EX-UE 9	Extra 27
He Ding	EX-LE 2	Extra 38
Nei Xi Yan	EX-LE 4	–
Xi Yan	EX-LE 5	Extra 37
Lan Wei Xue	EX-LE 7	Extra 39
Ba Feng	EX-LE 10	Extra 40

Outline	Essentials	König/Wancura
Extra 6	Ex 4	PaM 1
Extra 1	Ex 1	PaM 3
Extra 3	Ex 3	PaM 6
Extra 2	Ex 2	PaM 9
–	–	PaM 30
Extra 17	Ex 6	N-P 45
Extra 21	Ex 7	PaM 85
Extra 19	–	PaM 75
–	–	PaM 108
Extra 28	Ex 16	PaM 107
Extra 31	–	PaM 156
–	–	PaM 145
Extra 32	–	PaM 145
Extra 33	Ex 18	PaM 142
Extra 36	Ex 20	PaM 137

○ EX-HN 1 "Si Shen Cong"
   "Mind Hearing"

Location: Si Shen Cong consists of four points which lie 1 Cun frontal, dorsal, and lateral, respectively, to Point GV 20.

Depth of needling: Each point is needled 0.5 to 1 Cun subcutaneously in direction GV 20.

Indication: Restlessness, nervousness (sedative effect like Point GV 20), vertigo, headache, insomnia; enhancing the effect of Point GV 20.

Combination with other points:
Insomnia:
EX-HN 1 + H 7 + Sp 6.
Nausea, Vomiting:
EX-HN 1 + P 6 + St 36.

Action in TCM: Subdues interior Wind.

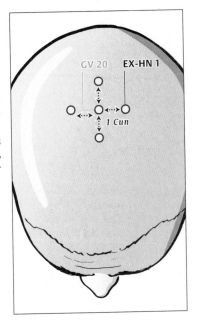

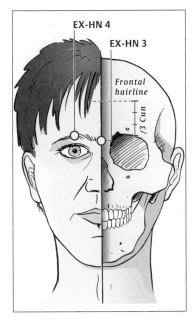

EX-HN 4

EX-HN 3

Frontal hairline

/3 Cun

pushed forward without inflicting discomfort.

Indication: Headache, especially frontal and tension headache, eye disorders, rhinitis, sinusitis, insomnia.

In the French literature, Yin Tang is called PdM (Point de Merveille). This refers to the quick action this point has on rhinitis and headache. For the "ventral magic triangle," see below.

Combination with other points: According to *J. Bischko*, the Point Yin Tang (EX-HN 3) and the two B 2 Points form the "ventral magic triangle." The ventral magic triangle acts relaxing, especially in case of headache, rhinitis, and sinusitis. The B 2 Points are needled perpendicularly, or with the tip of the needle directed toward the root of the nose (in the same direction as Point EX-HN 3).

Action in TCM: Eliminates Wind, calms the Mind (Shen), relieves the nose.

○ EX-HN 4 "Yu Yao"
    "Fish Spine"

Location: In the middle of the eyebrow, above the pupil when looking straight ahead.

Depth of needling: 0.5 Cun, subcutaneously toward the medial or lateral end of the eyebrow.

Indication: Eye disorders, frontal headache, facial paresis, trigeminal neuralgia.

Action in TCM: Purges Liver Fire, improves vision, alleviates pain and spasms.

○ EX-HN 3 "Yin Tang"
    "Seal Hall"

Location: In the middle between the eyebrows.
J. Bischko localizes this point deeper at the root of the nose.

Depth of needling: Approx. 1 Cun, subcutaneously in caudal direction toward the root of the nose. After forming a skin fold over the glabella, the needle can be

○ EX-HN 5 "Tai Yang"
"Greater Yang"

Location: In a depression approx. 1 Cun posterior to the middle of the connecting line between the lateral end of the eyebrow and the outer corner of the eye.

Depth of needling: Approx. 0.5 Cun, perpendicularly or subcutaneously toward the temple.

!
● There is usually a distinct palpable depression. Patients like to press this point themselves in case of headache. If pressure is a pleasant sensation, local therapy of acute headache is possible just by treating Tai Yang. (Otherwise take distal points in the case of acute headache.)

Indication: Headache, especially migraine, eye disorders, trigeminal neuralgia, facial paresis.

Action in TCM: Expels Wind, cools Heat, clears head and eyes, alleviates pain.

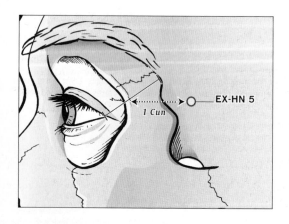

1 Cun

EX-HN 5

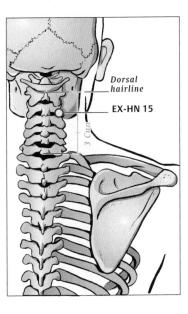

EX-HN 15 "Jing Bai Lao"
"Neck Labors"

Location: 2 Cun cranial to the tip of the spinous process of C7 and 1 Cun lateral to the median line.

> **!** The distance between the dorsal hairline and lower edge of spinous process of C7 measures 3 Cun.

Depth of needling: 0.5 to 1 Cun, in slightly caudal direction.

Indication: Cervical syndrome, spastic torticollis, fixed torticollis.

Action in TCM: Harmonizes the flow of Qi, removes obstructions from the meridian, expels Wind and Dampness.

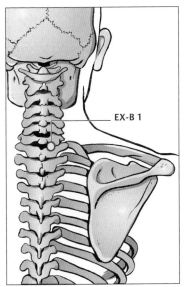

EX-B 1 "Ding Chuan"
"Stopping Asthma"

Location: 0.5 Cun lateral to Point GV 14 (lateral to the tip of the spinous process of C7).

Depth of needling: 0.5 to 1 Cun, in the direction of the spinal column, or in slightly caudal direction.

Indication: Disorders of the respiratory tract.

Action in TCM: There is no significant sphere of actions known.

○ EX-B 2 "Hua Tuo Jia Ji"
"Back-Filling Points" According to Hua Tuo

Location: This is a series of 17 points on each side of the spinal column, 0.5 Cun lateral to the tip of the spinous processes of T1 to L5. The points, therefore, lie at the same level as the points of the interior branch of the Bladder Meridian.

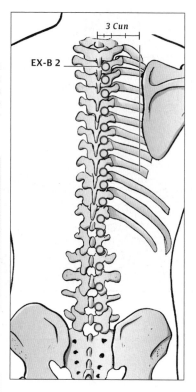

! The Hua Tuo Points lie in the region of the small vertebral joints (facet joints). This explains their effect on dysfunctions in this region. In the case of dysfunction in the cervical area, pressure-sensitive sites can be found along the line of Hua Tao Points also in cervical direction. These sites represent myogeloses in the area of paravertebral back muscles; they develop as a result of segmental dysfunctions and should be treated.

Depth of needling: 0.3 to 0.5 Cun, obliquely against the vertebrae.

! When needling the points of the interior branch of the Bladder Meridian at an angle of 45° in median direction, the needle tips reach the area of the Hua Tuo Points, thus enhancing the effect.

Indication: Local pain in the region of the spinal column, chronic dysfunction of internal organs.

Action in TCM: There is no fundamental sphere of actions known.

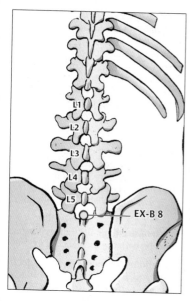

○ EX-B 8 "Shi Qi Zhui"
"Seventeenth Vertebra" (As Counted From T1)

Location: Below the tip of the spinous process of L5.

❗ Shi Qi Zhui lies in the region of the lumbar–sacral transition where instabilities, in particular, play a major role. Instability represents a contraindication to manipulation (the therapeutic approach of chiropractic); with acupuncture, however, treatment of dysfunctions with increased joint mobility (instability) and diminished joint mobility (blockage) is possible.

Depth of needling: Approximately 0.5 Cun, obliquely in cranial direction into the area of the interspinal ligament (for details on depth of needling, see Point GV 4, p. 97).

Indication: Lumbago, lumbago–sciatica syndrome, disordered menstruation, vaginal hemorrhage, pelvic presentation during pregnancy: combination with Point B 67 (moxa).
Caution! There is a risk of triggering uterine contractions!

Action in TCM: There is no fundamental sphere of actions known.

○ EX-UE 8 "Wai Lao Gong"
 "Exterior Pericardium 8"
 Also known as "Luo Zhen"
 "Outer Laogong"

Location: On the back of the hand, at the transition between the body and head of metacarpal bones II and III, approx. 0.5 Cun proximal to the metacarpophalangeal joints II and III.

Depth of needling: 0.5 to 1 Cun, obliquely in proximal direction, or perpendicularly.

Indication: Cervical syndrome, pain in the neck, pain in the shoulder.
Remark: According to *König/Wancura*, Point PaM 108 has the same localization as Luo Zhen. Point PaM 108 is an important distal point for acute cervical syndrome and/or pain in the shoulder.

Action in TCM: Harmonizes the flow of Qi and Blood, removes obstructions from the meridian, alleviates pain.

○ EX-UE 9 "Ba Xie"
 "Eight Pathogenic Factors"

Location: Four points on the back of each hand.
With the fist clenched loosely, the points are found proximal to the end of the folds between the fingers, at the border between red and white skin.

> **!** Localization of the metacarpophalangeal joints is best accomplished by mild traction of the respective finger. This causes the skin in the joint area to be slightly drawn inside.

Depth of needling: 0.3 Cun, in proximal direction with the fist clenched loosely.

Indication: Affections of the metacarpophalangeal joints, headache, toothache, restlessness, osteoarthritis and arthritis in the fingers.

Action in TCM: Expels exterior pathogenic factors.

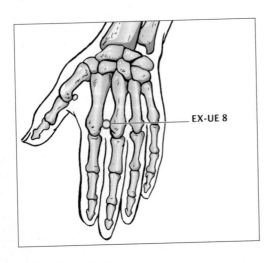

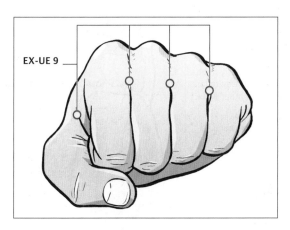

EX-UE 9

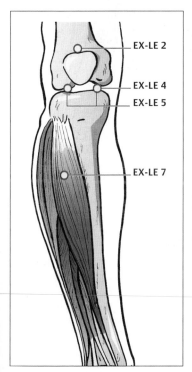

EX-LE 2
EX-LE 4
EX-LE 5
EX-LE 7

○ **EX-LE 2 "He Ding"**
"Crane Crown"

Location: In the middle of the upper edge of the patella.

Depth of needling: Approx. 0.3 Cun, perpendicularly.
Advice: When needling very deeply, there is a risk of puncturing the suprapatellar bursa and causing an infection.

Indication: Pain and dysfunction in the knee (wobbly knee, involuntary giving way of the knee).

Combination with other points:
Gonalgia: EX-LE 2 + St 36 + GB 34 + Sp 9.

Action in TCM: There is no fundamental sphere of actions known.

○ **EX-LE 4 "Nei Xi Yan"**
"Inner Knee-Eye"
(EX-LE 4 is part of EX-LE 5)

Location: When the knee is slightly bent, in the depression medial to the patellar ligament in the region of the inner Knee Eye.

Depth of needling: 0.3 Cun, perpendicularly, or approximately 0.5 Cun subcutaneously in the direction of Point St 35 (see Point EX-LE 5).

Indication: Gonalgia.

Action in TCM: There is no fundamental sphere of actions known.

○ **EX-LE 5 "Xi Yan"**
"Knee-Eyes"

Location: A pair of points below the patella, medial and lateral to the patellar tendon, namely the Points St 35 and EX-LE 4. Hence, Point EX-LE 4 is included in EX-LE 5.

! These two points correspond to the puncture sites for arthroscopy. When needling deeply, the needle may end up in an intra-articular position. (Caution! This is undesirable.)

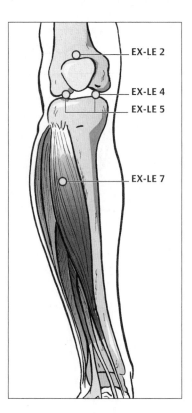

Depth of needling: 0.3 Cun, perpendicularly (see also Point EX-LE 4).

Indication: Pain and dysfunction in the knee (see Point EX-LE 2).

Combination with other points: Gonalgia: EX-LE 5 + EX-LE 2 + St 36 + GB 34 + Sp 9.

Action in TCM: There is no fundamental sphere of actions known.

○ **EX-LE 7 "Lan Wei Xue"**
"Appendix Point"

Location: On the Stomach Meridian, 2 Cun distal to St 36.

Depth of needling: 1 to 1.5 Cun, perpendicularly.

Indication: Test point for appendicitis (important for diagnosis), pain and dysfunction in the leg.

Action in TCM: There is no fundamental sphere of actions known.

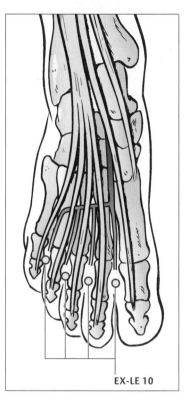

EX-LE 10

○ **EX-LE 10 "Ba Feng"**
  "Eight Winds"

Location: Four points on the back of the foot, proximal to the end of the interdigital creases, at the border between red and white skin.

> **!** Localization of the metacarpophalangeal joints is best accomplished by mild traction of the respective toes. This causes the skin in the joint area to be slightly drawn inside.

Depth of needling: Approximately 3 Cun in slightly proximal direction.

Indication: Pain in the back of the foot.

Action in TCM: Expels exterior pathogenic factors (especially Wind), relaxes the tendons, removes obstructions from the meridian, alleviates pain.

Part 2:
Ear Acupuncture Points

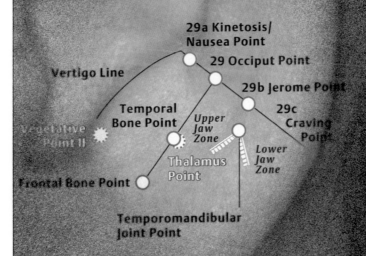

Point Zero

29a Kinetosis/
Nausea Point

29 Occiput Point

Vertigo Line

29b Jerome Point

Temporal
Bone Point

Upper
Jaw
Zone

29c
Craving
Point

Vegetative
Point II

Lower
Jaw
Zone

Thalamus
Point

Frontal Bone Point

Temporomandibular
Joint Point

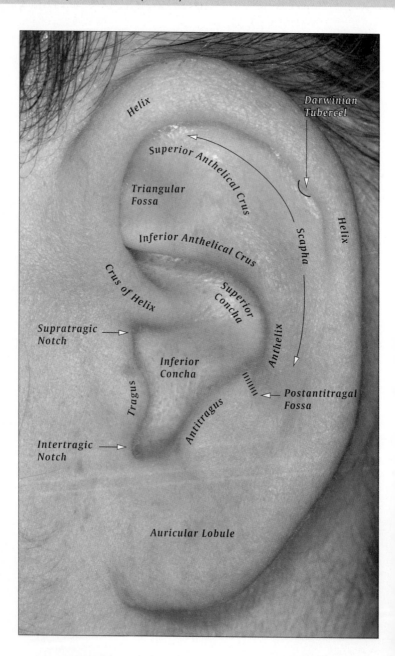

The outer shape of the auricula is formed by the helical brim (helix). The helix originates on the floor of the concha and ascends as the root of helix (crus of helix). It is followed by the body of the helix which descends as the tail of the helix toward the ear lobe. The helix then turns into the ear lobe (auricular lobule). In the upper part of the helix, we usually find a protrusion or widening of the helical brim, the darwinian tubercle (auricular hillock).

Parallel to the helix runs the anthelix. It originates in the cranial part of the auricula with two legs, the inferior anthelical crus and the superior anthelical crus. Between the two anthelical crura lies the triangular fossa. The anthelix turns into the antitragus in the lower part of the ear. The border between them is formed by the postantitragal fossa. Between the helix and the superior anthelical crus plus anthelix lies the scapha.

The tragus is bordered by the intertragic notch and the supratragic notch.

At the bottom of the auricula lies the cavity of concha. The concha is divided by the ascending crus of helix into two parts, the superior concha (cymba) and the inferior concha.

The outer auditory canal (external acoustic meatus) lies in the inferior concha and is covered from view by the tragus.

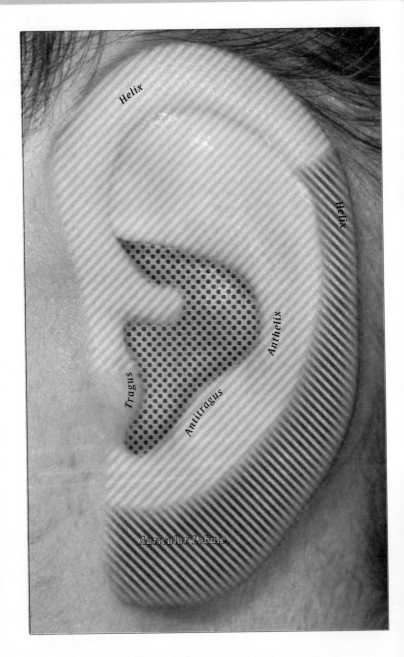

The auricula is innervated by three nerves:

▶ the auricular branch of the vagus nerve,
▶ the auriculotemporal nerve of the trigeminal nerve,
▶ the great auricular nerve of the cervical plexus.

The auricular branch of the vagus nerve innervates the concha. The "endodermal organs" are projected here. The great auricular nerve of the cervical plexus supplies the lobule, the outer helical brim up to approximately the darwinian tubercle, and the back of the ear. These areas correspond to the ectodermal germ layer.

The remaining, and by far the largest, part of the ear is innervated by the auriculotemporal nerve of the trigeminal nerve. The "mesodermal organs" are projected here.

According to *Nogier*, the different zones are assigned to different functional areas: the endodermal zone to the metabolism, the mesodermal zone to the motor system, the ectodermal zone to the head and central nervous system.

In line with this tripartition, *Nogier* found one control point for each functional area; these are the Omega Points.

The description of the auricular zones of

Auriculotemporal nerve
of trigeminal nerve

Auricular branch
of vagus nerve

Great auricular nerve
of cervical plexus

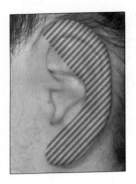

◀ Cervical plexus

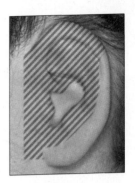

Trigeminal nerve ▶

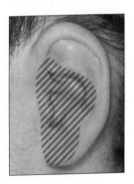

◀ Intermediate nerve
(facial nerve)

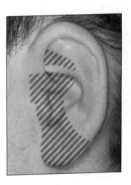

Glossopharyngeal nerve ▶

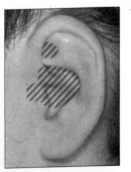

◀ Vagus nerve

innervation and the various somatotopic presentations according to the Russian school goes back to *R. A. Durinjan*. The first comprehensive German-language presentation of Russian auriculotherapy came from *R. Umlauf* and was published in 1988 in the German journal of acupuncture, *Deutsche Zeitschrift für Akupunktur*.

According to *Durinjan*, the following five nerves participate in the innervation of the auricula:

▶ fibers of the cervical plexus,
▶ the trigeminal nerve,
▶ the intermediate nerve of the facial nerve,
▶ the glossopharyngeal nerve,
▶ the auricular branch of the vagus nerve.

The innervation zones show distinct overlaps of the areas innervated by the five participating nerves. No auricular zone is exclusively innervated by one single nerve. This might explain why two or more acupuncture points of different functions are projected on identical anatomical sites.

Likewise, projections of the same organ are ascribed to different sites of localization. For example, we find projections which correspond to the parenchyma of the organ, next to them projections of the corresponding nervous innervation, and, finally, projections representing the functional state of the organ.

Due to the variation in auricular shape, it is conceivable that the overlaps of innervation zones also vary individually. Thus, the frequently described points are really zones rather than points in which the actual ear acupuncture point must be searched for according to individual circumstances. No doubt, this approach goes back to *Nogier* who tried to find individual representations of acupuncture points by means of the auriculocardiac reflex (ACR).

Nogier's Reflex (ACR, Auriculocardiac Reflex)

Underlying Nogier's reflex is a cutaneovascular reflex discovered by *Nogier* in 1968. He noticed a change in the pulse wave of the radial artery when stimulating irritated ear points or zones. While doing so, he observed two phenomena: an increase in pulse strength, which he called positive ACR, and a decrease in pulse strength, which he called negative ACR.

A positive ACR indicates an irritated zone in need of treatment.

For the school of *Nogier*, this is the most important approach when selecting acupuncture points. In this aspect, the school of auriculomedicine differs significantly from the Chinese school.

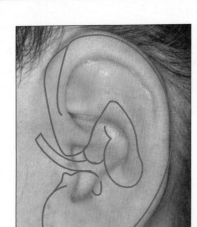

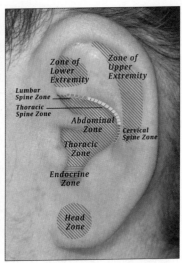

Zone of
Lower
Extremity

Zone of
Upper
Extremity

Lumbar
Spine Zone

Thoracic
Spine Zone

Abdominal
Zone

Cervical
Spine Zone

Thoracic
Zone

Endocrine
Zone

Head
Zone

The distribution of ear acupuncture points on the auricula follows a certain pattern. Localization of individual organs or body regions corresponds to that in an inverted fetus:

▶ The points in the area of the ear lobe are related to the head and face.
▶ The upper extremity is projected in the area of the scapha.
▶ The points on the anthelix and anthelical crura are related to the trunk of the body and the lower extremity.
▶ The internal organs are projected in the concha.
▶ According to *Nogier*, the lower extremity is projected in the triangular fossa; according to the Chinese school, the pelvic organs are projected here.
▶ According to *Nogier*, the sympathetic innervation of the intestine is projected on the crus of helix. The Chinese school assigns this area to the diaphragm.
▶ The points related to hormonal activity are also assigned differently: The Chinese school describes only an endocrine region, while *Nogier* differentiates between hypothalamic projections of the adrenal gland, thyroid gland, parathyroid gland, and mammary gland.

These slightly different anatomical circumstances are not contradictory; they may be understood as different reaction sites. We can distinguish here between functional and special pathological disorders. Nogier's points can often be assigned to organ-specific pathologies, while the Chinese school describes more the functional relationships. According to *Nogier*, the motor elements are projected on the back of the auricula and the sensory elements on the front of the auricula. Thus, the motor zone of an organ on the back of the ear is located exactly opposite to the sensory zone of that organ on the front of the ear.

Important:
Depending on the affiliation with one or the other school, the localization of individual points may vary significantly. This must be seen from the angle that ear acupuncture points are in fact zones in which each active point must then be localized.

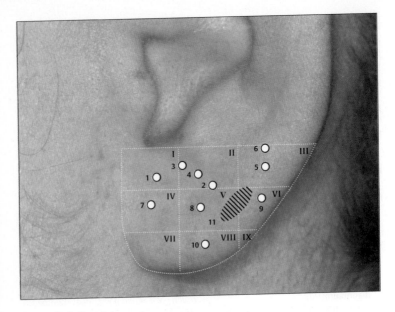

How to find the points:

We can divide the lobule into nine fields by drawing three horizontal and two vertical lines and using the natural border of the ear lobe. Inside these fields we find the 11 acupuncture points of the lobule.

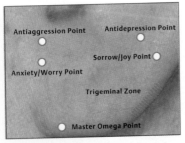

For comparison: Important points on the lobule according to Nogier.

Zone of Anxiety and Worry
Zone of Sorrow and Joy
Antidepression Point
Antiaggression Point
Master Omega Point
Trigeminal Zone

○ **1 Analgetic Point for Tooth Extraction**

Location: Quadrant I.

Indication: Analgesia for tooth extraction.

○ **2 Roof of Mouth Point**
(Upper Palate Point)

Location: Quadrant II.

Indication: Trigeminal neuralgia, toothache.

○ **3 Floor of Mouth Point**
(Lower Palate Point)

Location: Quadrant II.

Indication: Trigeminal neuralgia, toothache.

○ **4 Tongue Point**

Location: Quadrant II.

Indication: Stomatitis, toothache.

○ **5 Upper Jaw Point**

Location: Quadrant III.

Indication: Trigeminal neuralgia, toothache.

○ **6 Lower Jaw Point**

Location: Quadrant III.

Indication: Trigeminal neuralgia, toothache.

○ **7 Analgetic Point for Toothache**

Location: Quadrant IV.

Indication: Stomatitis, toothache.

○ **8 Eye Point**

Location: Quadrant V.

Indication: Inflammatory eye disorders, hordeolum, glaucoma, cephalalgia that radiates into the eyes.

○ **9 Inner Ear Point**

Location: Quadrant VI.

Indication: Vertigo, tinnitus, impaired hearing.

○ **10 Tonsil Point**

Location: Quadrant VIII.

Indication: The point has lymphatic activity.

○ **11 Cheek Zone**

Location: Quadrant V/VI.

Indication: Facial paresis, trigeminal neuralgia.

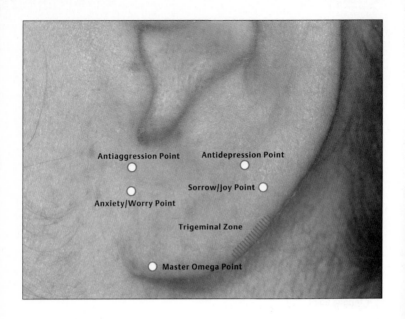

- Antiaggression Point
- Antidepression Point
- Sorrow/Joy Point
- Anxiety/Worry Point
- Trigeminal Zone
- Master Omega Point

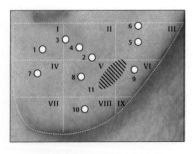

For comparison: Points on the lobule according to Chinese nomenclature.

1 Analgesia Point for Tooth Extraction
2 Roof of Mouth Point
3 Floor of Mouth Point
4 Tongue Point
5 Upper Jaw Point
6 Lower Jaw Point
7 Analgesia Point for Toothache
8 Eye Point
9 Inner Ear Point
10 Tonsil Point
11 Cheek Zone

◯ Zone of Anxiety and Worry

Location: Below the Antiaggression Point.

Indication: Anxiety, worry.

> **!** **In case of right-handedness:** Anxiety is treated on the right ear; worry is treated on the left ear.
> **In case of left-handedness:** vice versa.

◯ Antidepression Point

Location: On the extension of the Vegetative Groove, on a horizontal line with the Antiaggression Point.

Indication: Depressive mood.

◯ Antiaggression Point

Location: At the lower edge of the intertragic notch, toward the face.

Indication: An important psychotropic point. Addiction treatment.

◯ Master Omega Point

Location: On the caudal part of the lobule toward the face, on an imaginary line running vertically through the very tip of the tragus.

Indication: An important psychotropic point; intensely effective, harmonizes the vegetative system.

◯ Trigeminal Zone

Location: On the lateral edge of the lobule, middle to lower third.

Indication: Trigeminal neuralgia.

◯ Zone of Sorrow and Joy

Location: On the occipital part of the lobule, at the same level as the Zone of Anxiety and Worry.

Indication: Impaired joy of life, sorrow.

> **!** **In case of right-handedness:** Impaired joy of life is treated on the right ear; sorrow is treated on the left ear.
> **In case of left-handedness:** vice versa.

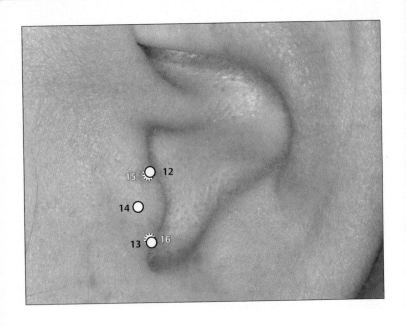

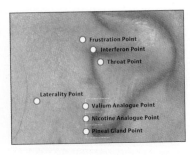

For comparison: Important points on the tragus and supratragic notch according to Nogier and Bahr.

Frustration Point
Interferon Point
Throat Point
Laterality Point
Valium Analogue Point
Nicotine Analogue Point
Pineal Gland Point

12 Apex of Tragus Point

Location: On the cranial side of a single-peaked tragus. On the cranial peak of a double-peaked tragus.

Indication: Analgesia. The point has anti-inflammatory activity.

13 Adrenal Gland Point
(ACTH Point, According to Nogier)

Location: On the lower third of a single-peaked tragus. On the caudal peak of a double-peaked tragus.

Indication: Allergic diathesis, joint disorders, chronic inflammation, functional circulatory disorders, paresis, neuralgia.

14 External Nose Point

Location: In the middle of the base of the tragus.

Indication: Local afflictions of the nose (eczema, rhinophyma, etc.).

15 Larynx/Pharynx Point

Location: On the inside of the tragus at the level of Point 12.

Indication: Pharyngitis, tonsillitis.

▶ Caution! Danger of collapsing (vagus irritation).

16 Inner Nose Point

Location: On the inside of the tragus at the level of Point 13.

Indication: Rhinitis, sinusitis.

▶ Caution! Danger of collapsing (vagus irritation).

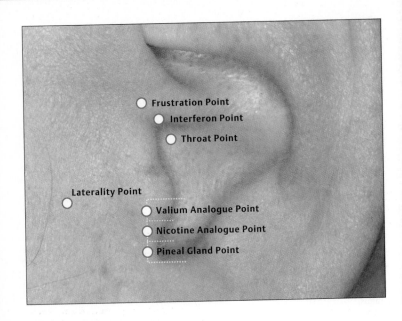

How to find the points:

A horizontal line through the middle of the tragus and another line through the bottom of the intertragic notch are connected by a vertical line roughly 3 mm in front of the tragus edge. The distance between the two lines is divided by three. In the middle of each subsection is located one of the following points: Valium Analogue Point, Nicotine Analogue Point, and Pineal Gland Point.

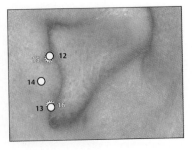

For comparison: Important points on the tragus according to Chinese nomenclature.

12 Apex of Tragus Point
13 Adrenal Gland Point
14 External Nose Point
15 Larynx/Pharynx Point
16 Inner Nose Point

○ **Frustration Point**

Location: In the groove between the tragus and crus of helix.

Indication: Psychosomatic afflictions.

○ **Interferon Point**

Location: In the corner of the supratragic notch.

Indication: The point has an immuno-modulating effect and anti-inflammatory activity.

○ **Throat Point**

Location: In the cranioventral part of the inferior concha.

Indication: Afflictions in the neck area, globus sensation, toothache.

○ **Laterality Point**

Location: On a horizontal line roughly 3 cm from the middle of the tragus.

▶ Preferred needling on the right side in case of right-handedness, on the left side in case of (masked) left-handedness.

Indication: Laterality dysfunction. The point strengthens the emotional balance through stress relief. Provides emotional stability in case of right–left oscillation, psychosomatic syndromes, and addiction treatment.

○ **Valium Analogue Point**

Location: On the descending part of the tragus (see "How to Find the Points," p. 130).

Indication: Addiction treatment. The point has general sedating activity.

○ **Nicotine Analogue Point**

Location: Just below the Valium Analogue Point (see "How to Find the Points," p. 130).

Indication: Addiction treatment.

○ **Pineal Gland Point**

Location: Below the Nicotine Analogue Point (see "How to Find the Points," p. 130).

Indication: Disturbed circadian rhythm. A psychotropic point of overriding importance; an adjuvant point in hormonal disorders.

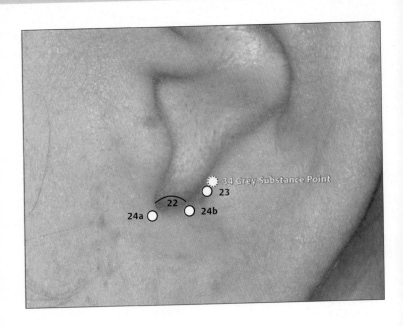

34 Grey Substance Point
23
22
24a
24b

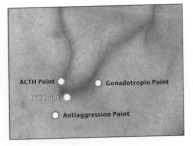

ACTH Point
Gonadotropin Point
TSH Point
Antiaggression Point

For comparison: Important points on the intertragic notch according to Nogier.
ACTH Point
Gonadotropin Point
TSH Point
Antiaggression Point

○ **22 Endocrine Zone**

Location: At the bottom of the intertragic notch, toward the face.

Indication: All endocrine disorders (gynecologic and rheumatoid disorders, allergies, skin disorders).

▶ According to *Nogier*, this zone corresponds to the points of the adrenal gland, thyroid gland, and parathyroid gland.

○ **23 Ovary Point
(Gonadotropin Point, According to Nogier)**

Location: On the ventral and outer ridge of the antitragus ("Eye of the Snake" when viewing antitragus and anthelix as a snake).

Indication: Ovarial dysfunction, period-related migraines and skin disorders.

○ **24a Eye Point 1
24b Eye Point 2**

Location: Below the intertragic notch.

Indication: Non-inflammatory eye disorders, possibly myopia, astigmatism, opticus atrophy.

○ **34 Grey Substance Point**

Location: On the inside of the antitragus above the Ovary Point.

Indication: The point has a harmonizing effect, antiphlogistic activity, analgetic activity.

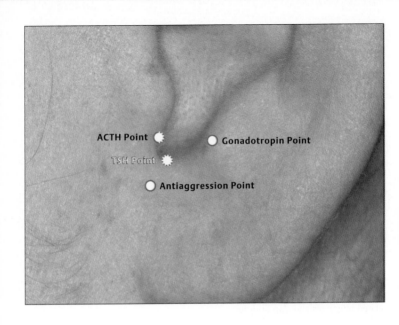

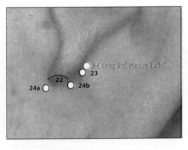

For comparison: Important points on the intertragic notch according to Chinese nomenclature.

22   Endocrine Zone
23   Ovary Point
24a Eye Point 1
24b Eye Point 2
34   Grey Substance Point

○ **ACTH Point**
(Adrenal Gland Point, According to
Chinese Nomenclature)

Location: On the caudal end to caudal third of the tragus, part on the inside.

Indication: An important point in the treatment of rheumatoid disorders, bronchial asthma, skin disorders.

○ **TSH Point**

Location: At the caudal edge of the intertragic notch, on the inside.

Indication: Thyroid-gland disorders, disorders of the urogenital tract, skin disorders, bulimia.

○ **Gonadotropin Point**
(23, Ovary Point, According to
Chinese Nomenclature)

Location: On the ventral and outer edge of the antitragus ("Eye of the Snake" when viewing antitragus and anthelix as a snake).

Indication: Sexual dysfunction, dysmenorrhea, amenorrhea.

○ **Antiaggression Point**

Location: Below the edge of the intertragic notch, toward the face.

Indication: An important psychotropic point. Addiction treatment.

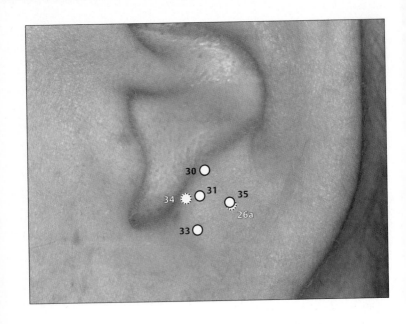

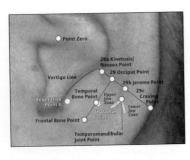

For comparison: Important points on the antitragus according to Nogier.

Postantitragal Fossa
29   Occiput Point
29a Kinetosis/Nausea Point
29b Jerome Point
29c Craving Point
Vertigo Line according to von Steinburg
Vegetative Point II (Grey Substance Point)
Thalamus Point
Temporal Bone Point
Frontal Bone Point
Temporomandibular Joint Point

○ **26a Pituitary Gland Point
(Thalamus Point, According to
Nogier)**

Location: On the inside of the antitragus, opposite Point 35.

Indication: A general analgetic point.

▶ According to *Nogier*, the point affects the homolateral body side.
▶ Caution! Contraindicated during pregnancy.

○ **30 Parotid Gland Point**

Location: On the tip of the antitragus.

Indication: Pruritus (strong antipruritic effect), inflammation of the parotid gland, mumps.

○ **31 Asthma Point**

Location: Between Points 30 and 33.

Indication: Bronchitis, asthma. The point affects the respiratory center.

○ **33 Forehead Point
(Frontal Bone Point, According to
Nogier)**

Location: On the ventral part of the antitragus.

Indication: Disturbances (-algia, -itis) in the forehead region, vertigo.

○ **34 Grey Substance Point
(Vegetative Point II, According to
Nogier)**

Location: On the inside of the antitragus, above the gonadotropin point (see p. 136, "Eye of the Snake").

Indication: The point has a harmonizing effect, antiphlogistic activity, and analgetic activity.

○ **35 Sun Point**

Location: In the middle of the base of the antitragus.

Indication: This point is frequently used in cephalgia, migraine, eye disorders, vertigo, insomnia.

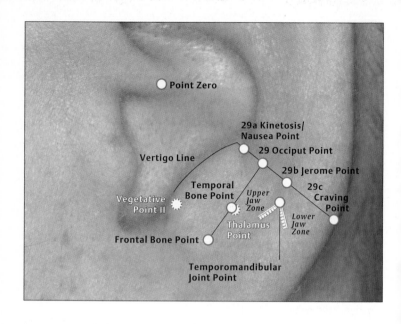

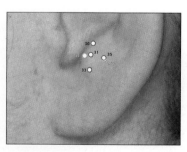

For comparison: Important points on the antitragus according to Chinese nomenclature.

26a Pituitary Gland Point
30 Parotid Gland Point
31 Asthma Point
33 Forehead Point
34 Grey Substance Point
35 Sun Point

Postantitragal Fossa

Location: A straight line is drawn from Point Zero through the notch between the antitragus and anthelix to the edge of the ear; it is called the Postantitragal Fossa. Important acupuncture points (29a, 29b, 29c) are located on this line.

Indication: For details, see the respective points.

29 Occipital Bone Point

Location: In the Postantitragal Fossa, midway between Points 29a and 29b. According to Chinese nomenclature, the localization of the Occiput Point is slightly more toward the face.

Indication: An important analgetic point with a broad spectrum of activity. Conditions of pain, skin disorders, functional circulatory disorders, allergies, vertigo, autonomic dysfunction, phase of recovery.

29a Kinetosis/Nausea Point

Location: Between the anthelical edge and Point 29 (Occiput Point).

Indication: Kinetosis, vomiting.

29b Jerome Point (Relaxation Point)

Location: In the Postantitragal Fossa, at the intersection with the Vegetative Groove.

Indication: For vegetative harmonization. Difficulty in falling asleep. In case of difficulty in staying asleep, the corresponding point on the back of the ear is needled.

29c Craving Point

Location: At the end of the Postantitragal Fossa, at the intersection with the edge of the ear.

Indication: Used within the scope of addition therapy.

Vertigo Line According to von Steinburg

Location: Along the Postantitragal Fossa and upper edge of the antitragus, slightly on the inside.

Indication: Vertigo.

Vegetative Point II

Location: On the inside of the antitragus, corresponding roughly to Point 34 (Grey Substance Point) of Chinese nomenclature.

Indication: The point has analgetic activity; vegetative harmonization.

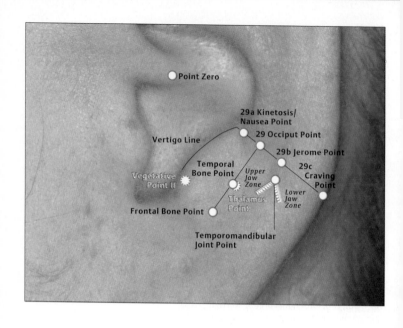

For comparison: Important points on the antitragus according to Chinese nomenclature.

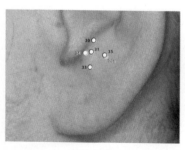

26a Pituitary Gland Point
30   Parotid Gland Point
31   Asthma Point
33   Forehead Point
34   Grey Substance Point
35   Sun Point

⊙ **Thalamus Point**
(26a, Pituitary Gland Point, According to Chinese Nomenclature)

Location: On the inside of the antitragus, opposite the Temporal Bone Point (Point 35, Sun Point).

Indication: A general analgetic point affecting the homolateral body side; vegetative harmonization. Premature ejaculation, frigidity.

▶ In case of articular rheumatism use gold needles.
▶ Caution! Contraindicated during pregnancy.

⊙ **Temporal Bone Point**
(35, Sun Point, According to Chinese Nomenclature)

Location: In the middle of the antitragus.

Indication: A frequently used point. Cephalalgia, migraine, eye disorders, vertigo, sleeping disorders.

⊙ **Frontal Bone Point**

⊙ **(33, Forehead Point, According to Chinese Nomenclature)**

Location: On the ventral part of the antitragus.

Indication: Disturbances (-algia, -itis) in the area of the forehead.

⊙ **Temporomandibular Joint Point**

Location: At the caudal end of the Vegetative Groove.

Indication: Disorders of the temporomandibular joint, cephalalgia.

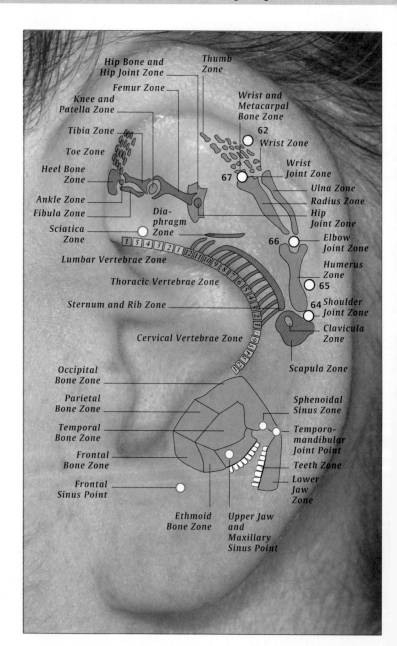

The cranial bones are projected on the area of the antitragus. Once again, there are some multiple projections. The frontal bone is represented on the ascending part of the antitragus. The ethmoid bone and the upper jaw are projected more toward the helical brim. The parietal bone is represented on the tip of the antitragus. The projection of the occipital bone forms the border in dorsal direction. The temporal bone is represented in the middle of the antitragus. The temporomandibular joint and the lower jaw with the teeth are projected next to the occipital bone.

The paranasal sinuses play a major role as field of disturbance. They are also projected in the antitragus region. The maxillary sinus is projected in the area of the upper jaw and the frontal sinus just below the area of the frontal bone. The sphenoidal sinus and the ethmoidal sinuses are projected on a line in the immediate vicinity of the maxillary sinus.

The upper extremity has its projection zones in the area of the scapha, while the lower extremity is projected in the triangular fossa.

64 Shoulder Joint Point (Chinese)

Location: Between C7 and the Vegetative Groove (approx. 4 mm medial to the groove).

Indication: Impingement syndrome, lateral/ventral pain in the shoulder.

65 Shoulder Point (Chinese)

Location: At the level of T3, medial to the Vegetative Groove.

Indication: Dorsal pain in the shoulder.

66 Elbow Point (Chinese)

Location: At the level of the lumbar spine projection zone, approximately 4 to 5 mm medial to the Vegetative Groove.

Indication: Epicondylitis, pain in the elbow.

67 Wrist Point (Chinese)

Location: On the elongation of the connecting line between Point Zero and T12, approximately 6 to 7 mm away from the Vegetative Groove.

Indication: Pain in the wrist, carpal tunnel syndrome.

62 Finger Points (Chinese)

Location: In the cranial scapha, caudal to the helical brim.

62 Thumb Point (Chinese)

Location: Immediately ventral to the Finger Points.

Indication: Used in pain therapy.

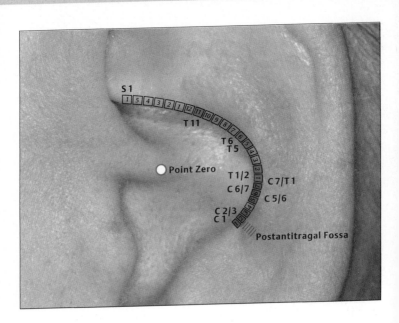

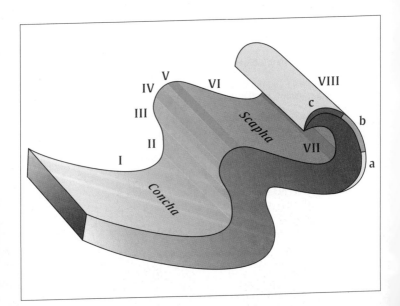

Nervous Organ Points of the Paravertebral Chain of Sympathetic Ganglia

○ **C1 (Superior Cervical Ganglion Point)**

Location: Zone II.

Indication: Tinnitus, vertigo.

○ **C2/3 (Middle Cervical Ganglion Point)**

Location: Zone II.

Indication: Functional heart complaints.

○ **C7/T1 (Inferior Cervical Ganglion Point, Stellate Ganglion Point)**

Location: Zone II.

Indication: Tinnitus, pain in the chest. Used for detecting fields of disturbance.

The Ear Relief in Cross Section (Zones I to VIII)

I	Zone of Organ Parenchyma
II	Zone of Paravertebral Chain of Sympathetic Ganglia
III	Zone of Nervous Control Points of Endocrine Glands
IV	Zone of Intervertebral Disks
V	Zone of Vertebrae
VI	Zone of Paravertebral Muscles and Ligaments
VII	Vegetative Groove (Zone of Origin of Sympathetic Nuclei)
VIII	Zone of Spinal Cord with projections of (a) motor tracts, (b) autonomic tracts, (c) sensory tracts

Nervous Control Points of Endocrine Glands

○ **T11 (Adrenal Gland Point)**

Location: Zone III.

Indication: Rheumatoid arthritis. This point has general anti-inflammatory and analgetic activities.

○ **T6 (Pancreas Point)**

Location: Zone III.

Indication: Indigestion.

○ **T5 (Mammary Gland Point)**

Location: Zone III.

Indication: Mastopathy, difficulties with breast-feeding.

○ **T1/2 (Thymus Gland Point)**

Location: Zone III.

Indication: Allergic disorders.

○ **C6/7 (Thyroid Gland Point)**

Location: Zone III.

Indication: Thyroid disorders, osteoporosis, fracture healing, cramps.

○ **C5/6 (Parathyroid Gland Point)**

Location: Zone III.

Indication: Bone diseases, osteoporosis, fracture healing, cramps.

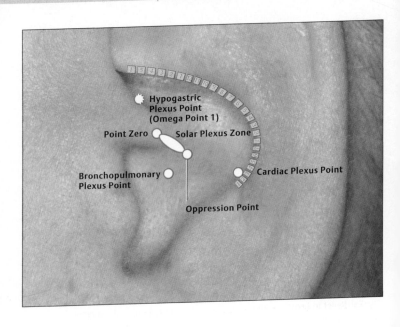

For comparison: Projection zones of internal organs according to Nogier.

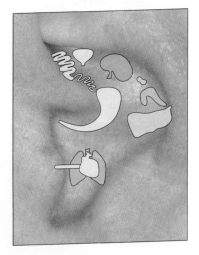

○ **Cardiac Plexus Point
(Wonder Point)**

Location: Ventral to the Middle Cervical Ganglion Point, at the level of C2/3.

Indication: Hypertension, functional heart complaints.

○ **Bronchopulmonary Plexus Point**

Location: In the inferior concha, ventral to the End Point of the Solar Plexus Zone (Oppression Point).

Indication: The point has broncholytic activity.

○ **Solar Plexus Zone**

Location: The zone including Point Zero (Point 82) and Oppression Point (Point 83).

Indication: Gastrointestinal complaints.

○ **Hypogastric Plexus Point
(Urogenital Plexus Point)**

Location: On the upper edge of the crus of helix, toward the superior concha, roughly in the middle between Point Zero and the intersection of the ascending helix and inferior anthelical crus. Identical with Omega Point 1.

Indication: Gastrointestinal and urogenital complaints, renal colic.

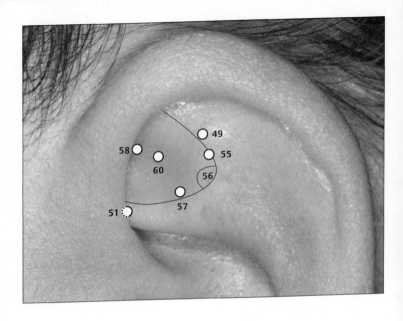

For comparison: Projection zones in the triangular fossa according to Nogier.

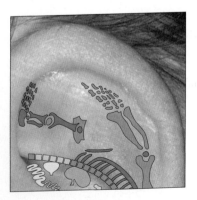

49 Knee Joint Point

Location: In the middle of the superior anthelical crus.

Indication: Pain in the knee area related to the function of the knee joint.

▶ The French Knee Point is located in the triangular fossa and represents the anatomy of the knee joint.

51 Autonomic Point (Sympathetic Point, Vegetative Point I)

Location: At the intersection of inferior anthelical crus and helix.

Indication: An important point; vegetative harmonization, vegetative stabilization of all visceral organs.

55 Shen Men Point (Divine Gate Point)

Location: Above the angle formed by the superior and inferior anthelical crura, more toward the superior anthelical crus.

Indication: One of the most important ear acupuncture points. Very effective for emotional stabilization; a point of overriding importance in conditions of pain; anti-inflammatory activity.

56 Pelvis Point

Location: In the angle formed by the superior and inferior anthelical crura.

Indication: Pain in the pelvic area.

▶ Hip Point and Pelvis Point according to Nogier are identical with Point 56.

57 Hip Point

Location: At the lower margin of the triangular fossa, ventral to the Pelvis Point (56).

Indication: Pain in the hip region.

58 Uterus Point

Location: In the triangular fossa, close to the helix.

Indication: Condition after uterus extirpation, e.g., postoperative pain.

60 Dyspnea Point

Location: Dorsal (and caudal) to the Uterus Point (58).

Indication: Bronchial asthma.

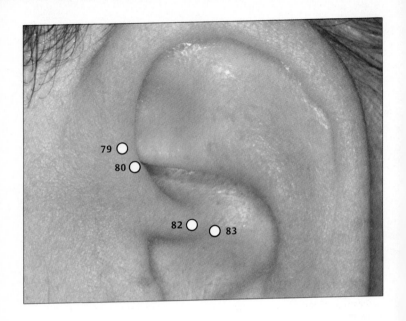

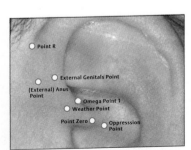

For comparison: Important points on the ascending helix according to Nogier.

Omega Point 2
Point R
External Genitals Point
(External) Anus Point
Omega Point 1
Point Zero
Oppression Point

○ **78 Allergy Point (Apex of Ear)**

Location: At the tip of the ear which forms upon folding the auricula.

Indication: Allergies; the point has an analgetic and emotionally harmonizing effect.

○ **79 External Genitals Point**

Location: On the ascending helix, at the level of the intersection with the inferior anthelical crus.

Indication: All forms of impotence; migraine, dysuria.

○ **80 Urethra Point**

Location: At the level of the intersection of the ascending helix and lower edge of the inferior anthelical crus.

Indication: Urinary-tract infection, dysuria.

○ **82 Diaphragm Point**

Location: On the ascending helix, cranioventral to the crus of the helix in a distinctly palpable fossula, corresponding to the topographic location of Point Zero of *Nogier*.

Indication: Hematological disorders. The point has spasmolytic activity.

▶ According to *Nogier*, this is the classic point of energy control.

○ **83 Bifurcation Point**

Location: At the origin of the crus of helix.

Indication: According to the Chinese school, the point does not play a major role.

▶ According to *Nogier*, End Point of the Solar Plexus Zone (Oppression Point).
▶ The point is often needled in states of anxiety.
Also called "Anxiety Point 2."

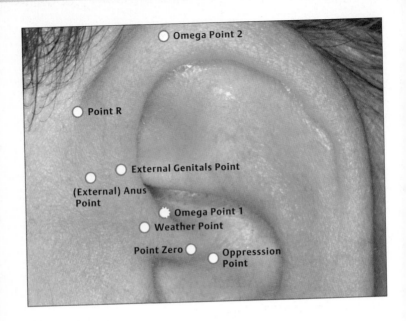

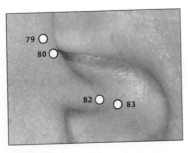

For comparison:
Important points on the helix according to Chinese nomenclature.

78 Allergy Point
79 External Genitals Point
80 Urethra Point
82 Diaphragm Point
83 Bifurcation Point

Omega Point 2

Location: On the upper edge of the helix, ventral to the Allergy Point (78) at the tip of the ear.

Indication: A point of overruling importance for the motor system; a point for disturbed relationships with the environment.

Point R (According to Bourdiol)

Location: On the ascending helix, in the fossula at the transition to the face.

Indication: An adjuvant point in psychotherapy.

External Genitals Point

Location: On the ascending helix, at the level of the inferior anthelical crus.

▶ Identical with Point 79 of the Chinese school.

Indication: All forms of impotence, migraine, dysuria.

(External) Anus Point

Location: On the ascending helix toward the face, at the level of the inferior anthelical crus.

Indication: Anal complaints, anal pruritus.

Omega Point 1

Location: At the upper edge of the crus of helix, in the inferior concha, roughly in the middle between Point Zero and the intersection of the helix and inferior anthelical crus.

Indication: Metabolic disorders, vegetative disorders, amalgam exposure.

Weather Point (According to Kropej)

Location: In the middle between the supratragic notch and the intersection of the inferior anthelical crus and helix.

Indication: Sensitivity to changes in the weather. An adjuvant point for angina pectoris and migraine, often detectable on the right ear.

▶ Relative contraindication in case of pregnancy.

Point Zero

Location: On the ascending crus of helix, cranioventral to its origin in a distinctly palpable fossula, corresponding to topographic location of Point 82 (Diaphragm) of the Chinese school.

Indication: According to *Nogier*, this is the classic point of energy control.

▶ Treatment with gold needles in case of psychovegetative exhaustion, treatment with silver needles in case of excessive needle reaction.

Furthermore, Point Zero has strong spasmolytic activity. In addition, hyperreflexia and hyporeflexia can be treated at this point on the auricula.

▶ Treatment with gold needles in case of hyperreflexia, with silver needles in case of hyporeflexia.

Oppression Point

Location: At the origin of the crus of helix (End Point of the Solar Plexus Zone), corresponding to Point 83 (Bifurcation Point) of the Chinese school.

Indication: According to *Nogier*, the End point of the Solar Plexus Zone is also called the Anxiety Point. Accordingly, its indications are: state of anxiety, functional gastrointestinal complaints.

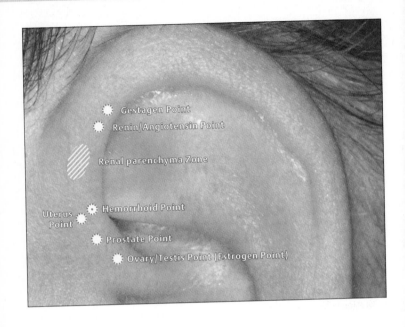

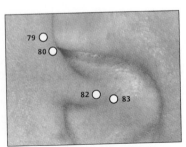

For comparison: Important points on the helix according to Chinese nomenclature.

79 External Genitals Point
80 Urethra Point
82 Diaphragm Point
83 Bifurcation Point

○ **Gestagen Point**

Location: Close to the fold of the ascending helix, on the inside, at the level of the superior anthelical crus.

Indication: Hormonal imbalance, hormone–related migraine.

○ **Renin/Angiotensin Point**

Location: Above the Renal Parenchyma Zone, on the inside.

Indication: Arterial hypertension (treatment with silver needle on the right ear), hypotension (treatment with gold needle on the right ear).

○ **Renal Parenchyma Zone**

Location: Inside of helical brim, roughly at the level of the triangular fossa.

Indication: Kidney diseases.

○ **Hemorrhoid Point**
  (Coccygeal Bone Point)

Location: On the end of the inferior anthelical crus (covered by helix).

Indication: Hemorrhoidal complaints, pain in the coccygeal region.

○ **Uterus Point**

Location: Roughly at the intersection of the inferior anthelical crus and the helix, on the inside.

Indication: Dysmenorrhea, field of disturbance after hysterectomy.

▶ Acupuncture of points on the ascending helix is contraindicated during pregnancy.

○ **Prostate Point**

Location: Between Ovary/Testis Point and Uterus Point, on the inside.

Indication: Prostatitis, prostate as field of disturbance.

○ **Ovary/Testis Point**
  (Estrogen Point)

Location: Slightly above the supratragic notch, inside the ascending helix, approximately 2 mm away from the reflection.

Indication: Hormonal dysfunction, hormone–related migraine.

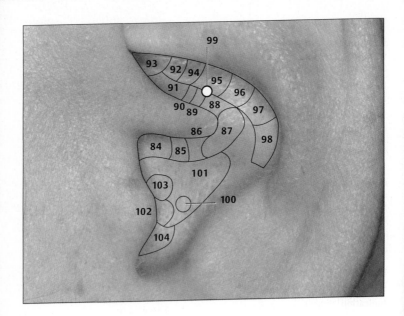

These points do not have a fixed localization but rather lie within a zone. The most sensitive point is used for needling.

▶ The points are needled according to their "meaning."
▶ Caution with points in the vicinity of the external acoustic meatus (danger of collapsing due to vagus irritation).

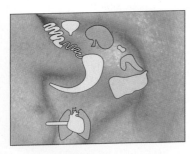

For comparison: Projection zones of internal organs according to Nogier.

84 Mouth Zone

Location: Inferior concha, close to the upper part of the supratragic notch.

Indication: Trigeminal neuralgia, stomatitis.

85 Esophagus Zone

Location: Inferior concha, below the middle of the ascending crus of helix.

Indication: Complaints in the esophageal region.

86 Cardia Zone

Location: Inferior concha, dorsal to the Esophagus Zone (85).

Indication: Stomach trouble, reflux.

87 Stomach Zone

Location: Surrounding the crus of helix.

Indication: Stomach trouble, gastritis, ulcer, nausea, vomiting.

88 Duodenum Zone

Location: Superior concha, above the crus of helix.

Indication: Gastrointestinal complaints.

89 Small Intestine Zone

Location: Superior concha, ventral to Duodenum Zone (88).

Indication: Gastrointestinal complaints.

90 Appendix Zone 4

Location: Superior concha, ventral to the Small Intestine Zone (89).

Indication: The point has lymphatic activity.

91 Large Intestine Zone

Location: Superior concha, opposite the Ureter Zone (94) and ventral to Appendix Zone 4 (90).

Indication: Gastrointestinal complaints, meteorism, obstipation, diarrhoea.

92 Urinary Bladder Zone

Location: Superior concha, cranial to the Large Intestine Zone (91).

Indication: Disorders of the urogenital tract, dysuria, incontinence.

93 Prostate Zone

Location: Superior concha, in the angle formed by the ascending helix and inferior anthelical crus.

Indication: Disorders of the prostate, dyssuria, impotence.

94 Ureter Zone

Location: Superior concha, dorsal to the Urinary Bladder Zone (92).

Indication: Dysuria.

▶ Often used in combination with the Kidney Zone (95).

95 Kidney Zone

Location: In the middle of the cranial part of superior concha.

Indication: One of the most important zones in ear acupuncture. It is used for disorders of the urogenital tract as well as joint disorders, menstrual complaints, migraine, insomnia, functional complaints and disorders of the ear, and also for addiction treatment.

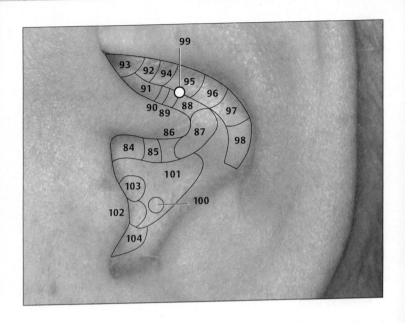

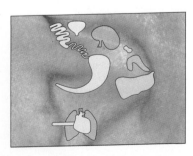

For comparison: Projection zones of internal organs according to Nogier.

96 Pancreas/Gall Bladder Zone

Location: Superior concha, dorsal to the Kidney Zone (95).

▶ According to Chinese localization, the gall bladder is projected on the right ear, the pancreas on the left ear. According to *Nogier*, the head of the pancreas is also projected on the right ear, while the body and tail are projected on the left ear.

Indication: Cholecystopathy, indigestion.

97 Liver Zone

Location: At the transition of the superior and inferior concha, craniodorsal to the Stomach Zone (87), close to the anthelix.

▶ On the right ear, the liver is projected in Zones 97 and 98, while its projection on the left ear is in Zone 97.

Indication: Gastrointestinal disorders, hematological disorders, skin disorders, eye disorders. An important zone used within the scope of addiction treatment.

98 Spleen Zone

Location: Inferior concha, caudal to the Liver Zone (97), close to the anthelix.

Indication: Indigestion, hematological disorders.

99 Ascites Point

Location: Superior concha, between Zones 88, 89, and 95.

Indication: An adjuvant point in liver disorders.

100 Heart Zone

Location: In the middle of the inferior concha.

Indication: Psychovegetative dysregulation, hypertension, hypotension, insomnia, anxiety, heart trouble, depression.

101 Lung Zone

Location: Inferior concha, surrounding the Heart Zone (100).

Indication: Disorders of the respiratory tract, skin disorders. Used within the scope of addiction treatment, especially during nicotine withdrawal.

102 Bronchial Zone

Location: Inferior concha, ventral to the Lung Zone (101), toward the external meatus.

Indication: Disorders of the respiratory tract.

103 Trachea Zone

Location: Inferior concha, above the Bronchial Zone (102).

Indication: Disorders of the respiratory tract.

104 Triple Warmer Zone

Location: Inferior concha, below the Bronchial Zone (102).

Indication: An adjuvant point in hormonal disorders.

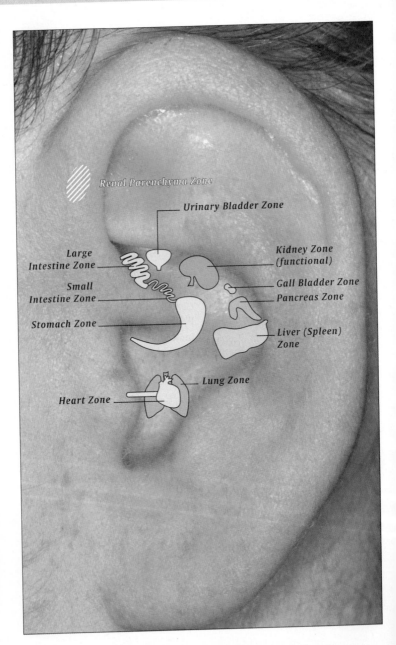

Renal Parenchyma Zone

Urinary Bladder Zone

Large
Intestine Zone

Kidney Zone
(functional)

Small
Intestine Zone

Gall Bladder Zone

Pancreas Zone

Stomach Zone

Liver (Spleen)
Zone

Lung Zone

Heart Zone

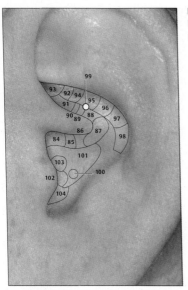

For comparison: Projection zones of the internal organs according to Chinese nomenclature.

84 Mouth Zone
85 Esophagus Zone
86 Cardia Zone
88 Duodenum Zone
89 Small Intestine Zone
90 Appendix Zone 4
91 Large Intestine Zone
92 Urinary Bladder Zone
93 Prostate Zone
94 Ureter Zone
95 Kidney Zone
96 Pancreas/Gall Bladder Zone
97 Liver Zone
98 Spleen Zone
99 Ascites Point
100 Heart Zone
101 Lung Zone
102 Bronchial Zone
103 Trachea Zone
104 Triple Warmer Zone

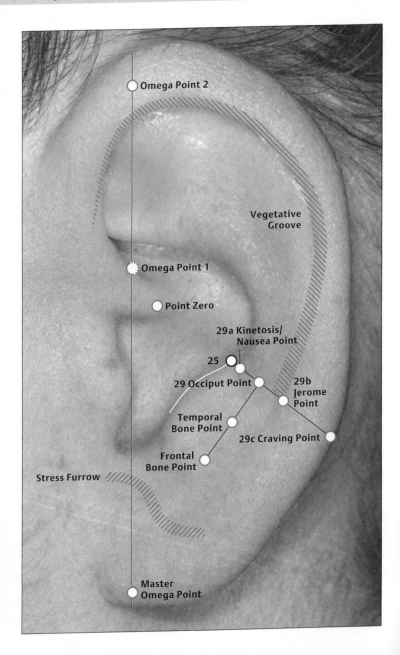

Several energy lines and treatment lines have been described on the auricula. Along the treatment lines are often found active acupuncture points. They usually form a basic framework when designing the individual treatment scheme.

Postantitragal Fossa

Location: A straight line is drawn from Point Zero through the notch between the antitragus and anthelix to the edge of the ear; it is called the Postantitragal Fossa. Important acupuncture points (29a, 29b, 29c) are located on this line.

Indication: For details, see the respective points.

⊙ 29a Kinetosis/Nausea Point

Location: At the transition of the antitragus to the anthelix, between Point 25 (Brain Stem Point, right on the edge of the anthelix at the transition of the antitragus to the anthelix) and Point 29 (Occiput Point).

Indication: Nausea, vomiting, and motion sickness.

⊙ 29 Occiput Point

Location: In the postantitragal fossa, midway between the Kinetosis/Nausea Point (29a) and Jerome Point (29b).

Indication: An important analgetic point, especially for cephalalgia.

⊙ 29b Jerome Point (Relaxation Point)

Location: In the Postantitragal Fossa, at the intersection with the Vegetative Groove.

Indication: An important point with a harmonizing effect on the vegetative system. Psychosomatic disorders, sexual dysfunction, insomnia.

▶ According to *Nogier*, needling of Point 29b is performed with gold needles in case of difficulty in falling asleep, and with silver needles in case of difficulty in staying asleep.

⊙ 29c Craving Point

Location: At the end of the Postantitragal Fossa on the helical brim.

Indication: Psychosomatic disorders, addiction treatment.

Sensory Line

Nogier calls the line between the Frontal Bone Point (33, Forehead Point), Temporal Bone Point (35, Sun Point) and Occipital Bone Point (29, Occiput Point) the Sensory Line. Energetic blood flow to the head is assigned to this line, as is the case with the body acupuncture point GV 16.

The Postantitragal Fossa and the Sensory Line represent two basic pillars in the treatment by ear acupuncture. The respective conspicuous points may be used together with the related spinal-column segment for basic therapy in pain treatment.

Stress Furrow

Location: This is a furrow running diagonally across the lobule. We find it often in patients who are under stress or cannot cope with stress in an appropriate manner. This furrow is of purely diagnostic importance. It has no therapeutic use.

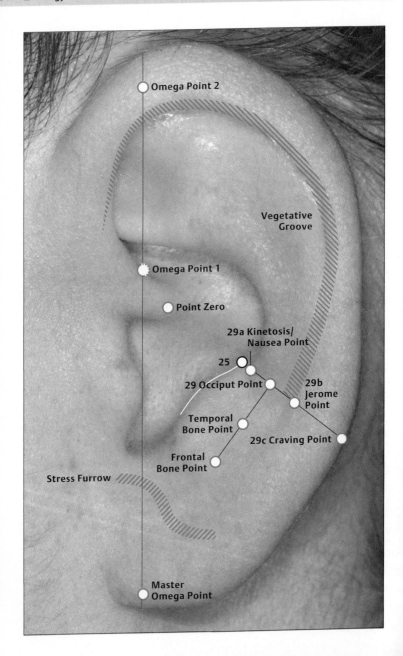

Vegetative Groove

Location: The Vegetative Groove runs cranially from the Postantitragal Fossa below the helical brim to the intersection of the inferior anthelical crus and ascending helix.

Indication: The Vegetative Groove represents an important treatment tool in ear acupuncture. It should be searched for active points prior to each treatment.

Line of Omega Points

This is the line connecting the three Omega Points according to *Nogier*. It runs vertically through the very tip of the tragus. *Nogier* divides the ear into three zones:

▶ the Endodermal Zone is assigned to metabolism,
▶ the Mesodermal Zone to the motor system,
▶ the Ectodermal Zone to the head and central nervous system and, therefore, to a higher level of regulation.

Corresponding to this tripartition, *Nogier* found a control point for each zone.

◯ Omega Point 2

Location: On the upper edge of the helix, ventral to the Allergy Point (78), on an imaginary line running vertically through the very tip of the tragus.

Sphere of action: Mesodermal Zone; area innervated by the auriculotemporal nerve of the trigeminal nerve.

Assignment: Motor system. A point for disturbed relationships with the environment.

◯ Omega Point 1

Location: On the upper edge of the crus of helix, roughly in the middle between Point Zero and the intersection of the ascending helix and inferior anthelical crus, on an imaginary line running vertically through the very tip of the tragus.

Sphere of action: Endodermal Zone; area innervated by the vagus nerve.

Assignment: Metabolism.

◯ Master Omega Point

Location: On the ventral lower part of the lobule, on an imaginary line running vertically through the very tip of the tragus.

Sphere of action: Ectodermal Zone; area innervated by the cervical plexus.

Assignment: Head and central nervous system.

Vertigo Line According to von Steinburg

Location: The line runs along the Postantitragal Fossa and on the inside of the antitragus; it is used in case of vertigo.

Indication: Vertigo.

Needle method: One should search for the most sensitive point or points on the line.

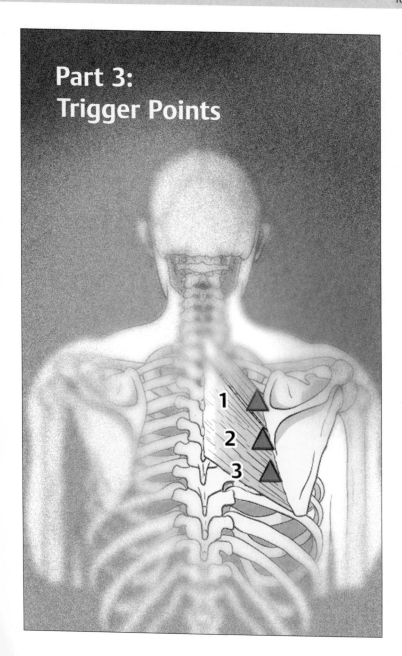

Part 3:
Trigger Points

Description of the Muscle

Origin: Deep lamina of temporal fascia, temporal plane, temporal fascia of sphenoid bone, back of zygomatic bone.

Insertion: Coronoid process of mandible, at its medial surface toward the third molar.

Innervation: Deep temporal nerves from the mandibular nerve (mandibular division of trigeminal nerve, third division of fifth cranial nerve).

Action: Closes the jaws;
posterior part: retracts lower jaw, supports chewing movements.

Miscellaneous: The superficial temporal artery runs on top of the muscle; it splits into parietal and frontal branch in the temporal area.

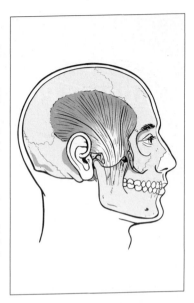

Trigger Points at the Temporal Muscle

Preliminary Remarks

There are four trigger-point areas in the temporal muscle which can be found on an imaginary line running toward the ear, beginning at the inferior part of the muscle at the level of the lateral corner of the eye. These trigger points are activated by faulty occlusion, direct traumas or long-term immobilization, but also by dental interventions or psychogenic factors (e.g., bruxism or pressing of the teeth), and less often by external climatic factors (e.g., draft or cold). Also to be considered are trigger points in the ipsilateral masseter muscle and in the contralateral temporal muscle. Less often involved are the medial and lateral pterygoid muscles, either unilaterally or bilaterally. Satellite trigger points appear as painful zones in the upper parts of the trapezius muscle and sternocleidomastoid muscle. The differential diagnosis should consider temporal arteriitis, polymyalgia rheumatica, and polymyositis.

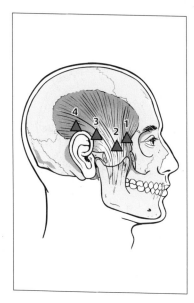

However, the typical pain projection areas which characterize the trigger points are absent in these conditions.

Examination of Trigger Points

The trigger point regions are palpated while the mouth is opened approximately 2 cm and the head is fixed. Local, pressure-sensitive indurations of the muscle with typical pain projection are present. The inside of the mandibular coronoid process is also examined by intraoral palpation. There are taut bands in the muscle where a brief local twitching of the muscle can be triggered (local twitch response).

Therapy of Trigger Points

While avoiding both branches of the temporal artery, the trigger points are needled in the conventional way, the needles remaining in place for 20 minutes. Alternatively, the shortened muscles can be directly relaxed by intramuscular stimulation with the acupuncture needle. As another option, trigger point infiltration with a local anesthetic in low concentration may be considered. This is followed by passive stretching of the muscle by pulling the lower jaw down and forward, using even postisometric relaxation if necessary.

Trigger Points and Areas of Pain Projection

▲ **Temporal Muscle, Trigger Point 1**

Located in the anterior part of the muscle, the point shows the following areas of pain projection: the incisors of the upper jaw, the lateral lower wing of the nose, the eyebrow, and the anterior part of the temporal bone.

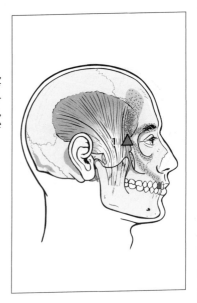

▲ **Temporal Muscle, Trigger Point 2**

Located in the anterior portion of the medial part of the muscle. Radiating symptoms are found in the region of the canine tooth and first premolar of the upper jaw. Further pain projections are found cranial to the trigger point.

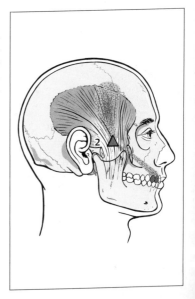

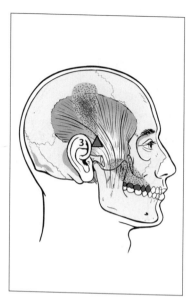

▲ **Temporal Muscle, Trigger Point 3**

Located in front of the auricula, the areas of pain projection lie in the molar region of the upper jaw and also run along the middle fibers of the temporal muscle above the zone of the trigger point.

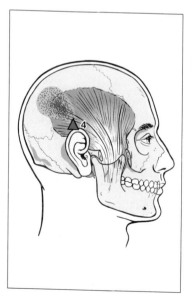

▲ **Temporal Muscle, Trigger Point 4**

Located behind the auricula, its area of pain projection runs along the dorsal fibers of the temporal muscle.

Important Acupuncture Points and Their Localizations

○ St 8

Location: 0.5 Cun from the frontal hairline toward the hair, in the angle of this hairline with the temporal hairline running perpendicular to it. Hence, the point lies 4.5 Cun lateral to acupuncture point GV 24.

○ EX-HN 5 (Extra 5, Tai Yang)

Location: Approximately 1 Cun toward the ear from the center of the line connecting the end of the eyebrow with the lateral corner of the eye.

○ St 7

Location: In the center of the depression below the zygomatic arch, i.e., in the mandibular notch between coronoid process and condylar process of the mandible.
The mandibular condyle can be easily palpated in front of the tragus (it slips forward when opening the mouth). In the depression just in front of it lies acupuncture point St 7. This point is searched for and needled when the mouth is closed.

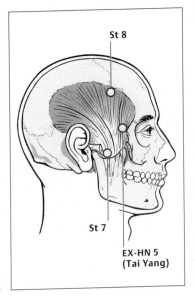

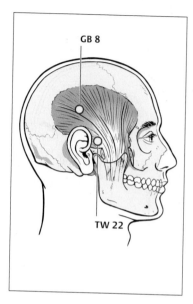

○ **TW 22**

Location: At the level of the auricular insertion, slightly ventral and cranial to acupuncture point TW 21, dorsal to the superficial temporal artery.

○ **GB 8**

Location: 1.5 Cun above the highest point of the auricula.

Gnathological Aspects of the Temporal Muscle, Anterior Part

Functional Aspects:
Adductor muscle (closes the mouth).

Palpation:
About 1 cm behind the lateral orbital margin.

Symptomatology:
Parietal headache,
central pressing of teeth,
near-central grinding of teeth.

Projected pain:
Pain in the medial and lateral incisors of the upper jaw (pulpal complaints, hyper-sensitivity, prolonged pain response to thermal stimuli), sometimes the sensation of pre-contact;
toward the temple,
from the temple through the upper jaw bone toward the incisors of upper jaw,
in parietal direction,
in supraorbital direction,
in retrobulbar direction.

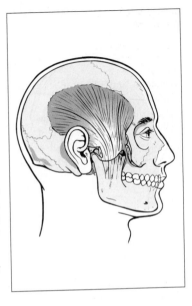

Gnathological Aspects of the Temporal Muscle, Medial Part

Functional aspects:
With the medial part alone: adductor muscle (closes the mouth),
together with the posterior part: retractor muscle.

Palpation:
Cranial to the ear.

Symptomatology:
Temporal headache,
occipital headache.

Parafunction:
Protrusion,
retrusion.

Projected pain:
Into the larynx,
toward the temple,
from the temple through the lateral upper jaw and the zygomatic arch toward the canine tooth and first premolar of upper jaw,
pain in the area of the canine tooth and first premolar of upper jaw (pulpal complaints, hypersensitivity, prolonged pain response to thermal stimuli), sometimes the sensation of pre-contact.

Gnathological Aspects of the Temporal Muscle, Posterior Part

Functional aspects:
Together with the medial part: adductor muscle (closes the mouth),
when supported by the medial part: retractor muscle.

Palpation:
Cranial to the ear.

Symptomatology:
Temporal headache,
occipital headache.

Parafunction:
Protrusion,
retrusion,
contributes to the displacement of the condyles leading to secondarily caused dysfunctions of the articular disk (dislocation of disk).

Projected pain:
Into the larynx,
toward the temple,
from the temple through the zygomatic arch into the lateral upper jaw, into the mucosa and into the molars,
pain in the area of the second premolar and molars of upper jaw (pulpal complaints, hypersensitivity, prolonged pain response to thermal stimuli), sometimes the sensation of pre-contact.

Description of the Muscle

Origin: Superficial part: lower border of lateral surface and temporal process of zygomatic bone;
deep part: lower border of medial surface of zygomatic arch.

Insertion: Superficial part: angle and ramus of mandible, toward the region of the second molars;
deep part: toward the upper third of ramus of mandible (masseteric tuberosity) and toward the base of the coronoid process.

Innervation: Masseteric nerve from the mandibular nerve (mandibular division of trigeminal nerve).

Action: Raises mandible, closes the jaws, supports protrusion.

Miscellaneous: The facial artery crosses the edge of the mandible at the anterior margin of the muscle.

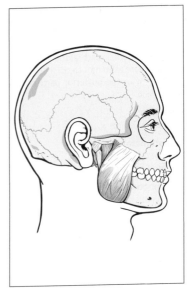

Trigger Points of the Masseter Muscle

Preliminary Remarks

A total of seven trigger points are distinguished within the masseter muscle, six of which are localized in the superficial part and only one in the deeper portion of the muscle. Bruxism, psychogenic factors, disturbed function of the temporomandibular joint (e.g., as a result of malocclusion), missing teeth, or poor jaw movement resulting from faulty position of the teeth may activate the trigger points. Acute traumas and acute strain can also contribute to activation. Frequently, however, the trigger points are activated through primary trigger points in the sternocleidomastoid muscle. Secondary trigger points are found in the temporal muscle and medial pterygoid muscle, and less often in the contralateral masseter muscle.

Examination of Trigger Points

With the mouth opened approximately 2 cm, examination of the trigger point regions is performed by pressing onto the trigger point zones while providing intraoral support. The typical projected pain can be triggered, and taut bands can be palpated within the muscle.

Therapy of Trigger Points

The trigger points are needled in the conventional way, the needles remaining in place for 20 minutes. Taut bands can be relaxed in a targeted way by means of intramuscular stimulation. If necessary, trigger point infiltration with a local anesthetic is also possible. This is followed by passive stretching of the muscle by pulling the upper jaw down and forward, which the patient then continues on his/her own.

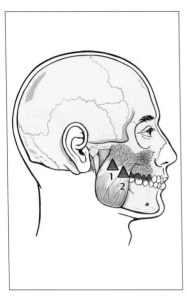

Trigger Points and Areas of Pain Projection

▲ Masseter Muscle, Trigger Points 1 and 2

Trigger points 1 and 2 are found in the superficial part of the muscle at the level of the upper-jaw teeth. Pain is projected into molars and premolars as well as into the upper jaw. Confusion with maxillary sinusitis is possible.

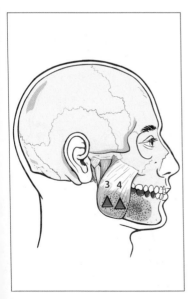

▲ Masseter Muscle, Trigger Points 3 and 4

Trigger points 3 and 4 are found at the level of the mandibular center. Pain is projected into the lower jaw in front of the masseter muscle and into the region of the premolars and molars of the lower jaw.

▲ Masseter Muscle, Trigger Points 5 and 6

Trigger points 5 and 6 are found right at the insertion of the superficial portion; areas of pain projection are the lower jaw bone, the eyebrow, and, facultatively, the region between the mandibular angle and ipsilateral eyebrow.

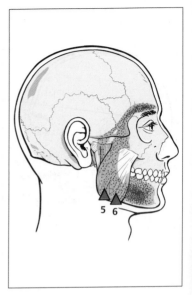

▲ Masseter Muscle, Trigger Point 7

Trigger point 7 is found right in front of the temporomandibular joint in the deep portion of the masseter muscle. Pain is localized over the temporomandibular joint and in the region of the inferior concha of the ear. A blunt pain is also present over the entire region of the masseter muscle.

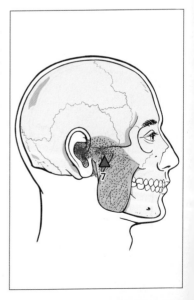

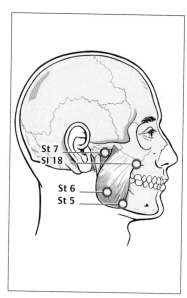

Important Acupuncture Points and Their Localizations

○ St 5

Location: Ventral to the mandibular angle at the anterior margin of the masseter muscle. Pulsation of the facial artery can be palpated here.

○ St 6

Location: Starting from the mandibular angle, acupuncture point St 6 lies approximately 1 Cun in craniofacial direction. The masseter muscle can be palpated here during biting.

○ St 7

Location: In the center of the depression below the zygomatic arch, i.e., in the mandibular notch between the coronoid process and condylar process of the mandible.
The mandibular condyle can be easily palpated in front of the tragus (it slips forward when opening the mouth). In the depression just in front of it lies acupuncture point St 7.

○ SI 18

Location: At the lower edge of the zygomatic arch, vertically below the outer corner of the eye, at the anterior margin of the masseter muscle.

Gnathological Aspects of the Masseter Muscle, Superficial Part

Functional aspects:
Adductor muscle (closes the mouth), protractor muscle

▶ supports mediotrusion when contracted on one side,
▶ supports protrusion when contracted on both sides.

Palpation:
During the relaxed state and when maximally contracted:

▶ at the origin below the zygomatic arch within the muscle belly,
▶ with two fingers at the insertion while the mouth is open, 1 cm cranial to the angle of the mandible at the aponeurosis,
▶ with both hands at the dorsal part of the body of mandible.

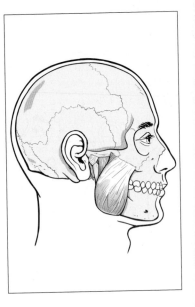

Symptomatology:
In case of severe pain: trismus (inability to open the mouth normally), bruxism, mainly in the protruding position

▶ at the canine tooth when contracted on one side,
▶ at the edge of the incisors when contracted on both sides.

Projected pain:
From the area of the premaxilla in retrobulbar direction and into the maxillary sinus (sinusitis–like symptoms), into the distribution areas of the infraorbital nerve and maxillary division of the trigeminal nerve, upper jaw (in the bone), mucosa of the lateral upper jaw.

Trigger point in the cranial part:
Pain in the second premolar, first and second molars of upper jaw (pulpal complaints, hypersensitivity, prolonged pain response to thermal stimuli).

Trigger point in the medial part:
Pain in the second premolar, first and second molars of lower jaw (pulpal complaints, hypersensitivity, prolonged pain response to thermal stimuli);
pain in the lower jaw in the region of the molars.

Trigger point in the lower part:
Pain radiating across the zygomatic arch and the anterior temporal area in suborbital direction toward the entire eyebrow and supraorbital arch;
in rare cases: unilateral tinnitus.

Description of the Muscle

Origin: Superior head: infratemporal fascia and infratemporal crest of greater wing of sphenoid bone;
inferior head: lateral surface of lateral pterygoid plate of sphenoid bone;
caudal head: between the two heads of the medial pterygoid muscle.

Insertion: Upper edge of the pterygoid pit of mandible, joint capsule and intra-articular disc of temporomandibular joint.

Innervation: Lateral pterygoid nerve from the mandibular nerve (mandibular division of trigeminal nerve).

Action: Lowers mandible, protrudes mandible, moves mandible from side to side.

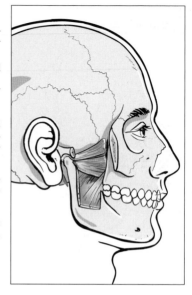

Trigger Points of the Lateral Pterygoid Muscle

Preliminary Remarks

There are two trigger points in this two-bellied muscle which rarely become manifest due to acute events (e.g., traumas), but usually as a result of chronic strain of the temporomandibular joint in case of malocclusion and in psychosomatic disorders (e.g., bruxism). Trigger points in this region rarely appear alone but rather in combination with trigger points of the masseter muscle and of posterior fibers of the temporal muscle.

Examination of Trigger Points

With the mouth opened approximately 3 cm, the muscle part close to the mandibular joint is palpated between the joint and zygomatic bone; with the mouth opened 5 to 8 mm and starting from the cheek, the muscle parts located further from the joint are palpated above the coronoid process of the mandible.

Therapy of Trigger Points

The following therapies may be considered: dry-needling, conventional acupuncture, and therapeutic local anesthesia. Reaching the muscle requires accurate anatomical knowledge. The trigger points are reached only at a depth of 3 cm. Stretching of the muscle is usually only possible with physiotherapeutic mobilization of the temporomandibular joint.

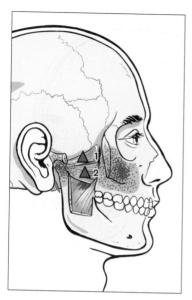

Trigger Points and Areas of Pain Projection

▲ **Lateral Pterygoid Muscle, Trigger Points 1 and 2**

The trigger point in the cranial part of the muscle is found below the zygomatic arch, the other one below the coronoid process of the mandible. The typical projection areas lie over the temporomandibular joint and at the level of the zygomatic arch.

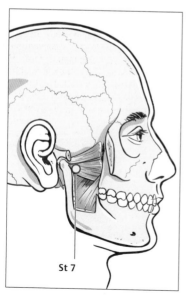

St 7

Important Acupuncture Point and Its Localization

○ **St 7**

Location: In the center of the depression below the zygomatic arch, i.e., in the mandibular notch between the coronoid process and condylar process of the mandible.

Gnathological Aspects of the Lateral Pterygoid Muscle

Functional aspects:
Bilateral activity: abductor muscle.
Unilateral activity: mediotrusion.

Palpation:
Can be performed only indirectly: behind the last molar, with the mouth opened half-way, between the maxillary tuber and lateral wing of the pterygoid process.

Symptomatology:
Indicator for the presence of parafunctions:

▶ frontal bruxism,
▶ eccentric bruxism.

Projected pain:
Pain in deep location,
into the ear,
into the temporomandibular joint,
into the tongue,
into the floor of the mouth,
into the maxillary sinus.

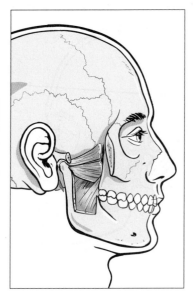

Description of the Muscle

Origin: Descending part: outer occipital protuberance to cervical vertebra C6; transverse part: spinous process of C7 to spinous process of thoracic vertebra T3; ascending part: vertebrae T3 to T12.

Insertion: Lateral third of clavicle, acromion and spine of scapula.

Innervation: Accessory nerve (11th cranial nerve).

Action: Broad range of movements in the shoulder region, among others: elevates shoulder (ascending part and descending part), retracts scapula medially (transverse part), and moves head when shoulder girdle is fixed (dorsal extension when contracted on both sides).

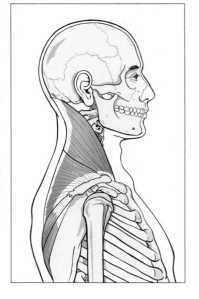

Trigger Points of the Trapezius Muscle

Preliminary Remarks

There are seven trigger points in the trapezius muscle. Activation of these trigger points results predominantly from chronic strain as a result of faulty posture during activities involving constant sitting, from scoliosis, as well as from physically unbalanced occupational activities (e.g., typing). Less often it results from acute traumas. In case of psychogenic stress, trigger points are especially common in this muscle. These trigger points are associated with those in the levator muscle of scapula or in the scalene muscles as well as in the sternocleidomastoid muscle and pectoral muscles.

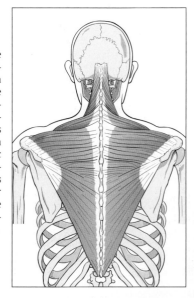

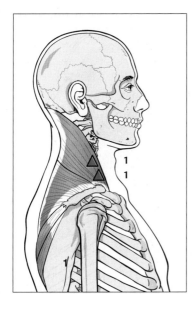

Examination of Trigger Points

The trigger points may be palpated either by using the thumb or by creating a forceps grip with the thumb and index finger. Apart from the triggered pain projections, a frequent characteristic feature is the appearance of shortened muscle structures where violent local twitch responses can be triggered. Examination of the patient is usually performed while the patient is sitting in round-back position and simultaneously grasping his/her upper arms with the opposite hands.

Therapy of Trigger Points

Conventional acupuncture, therapeutic local anesthesia, and intramuscular stimulation to loosen up the taut bands. Follow-up treatment by means of passive stretching of the muscular structures.

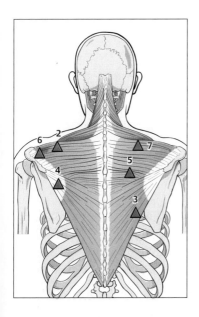

Trigger Points and Areas of Pain Projection

▲ Trapezius Muscle, Trigger Point 1

The area of trigger point 1 is found at the anterior margin of the clavicular part and leads to typical radiation toward the mastoid, mandibular angle, and into the area above the lateral eyebrow. Inconsistent pain projections between the tip of the mastoid process and the ascending part of the lower jaw, and also within a semicircular strip from the mastoid process via the occipital bone and temporal bone up to the temporal region.

▲ Trapezius Muscle, Trigger Point 2

Trigger point 2 is found in the transverse part at the transition from the medial third to the lateral third. Its main projection area lies dorsomedial to the mastoid process and extends in a weaker form from the trigger point to the main projection area.

▲ Trapezius Muscle, Trigger Point 3

Trigger point 3 is found 2 Cun medial to the medial margin of scapula at the level of the spinous process of T6. Its main area of pain projection extends into the region of the acromial and nuchal insertions of the muscle; the entire area of the muscle above the trigger point appears as secondary projection area.

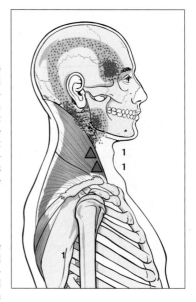

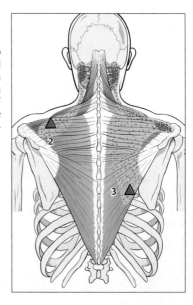

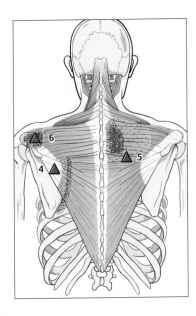

▲ Trapezius Muscle, Trigger Point 4

Trigger point 4 is localized 1 to 2 Cun lateral to the medial margin in a depression below the scapular spine and has its main area of pain projection at the medial margin of scapula.

▲ Trapezius Muscle, Trigger Point 5

Trigger point 5 is found just medial to the medial scapular margin, approximately 2 Cun above the scapular spine. The area of pain projection is localized between C6 and T3 immediately adjacent to the vertebrae and extends in a weakened form into the transverse part of the trapezius muscle.

▲ Trapezius Muscle, Trigger Point 6

Trigger point 6 is localized close to the insertion at the dorsal acromion, and here is also its area of pain projection.

▲ Trapezius Muscle, Trigger Point 7

The zone of trigger point 7 lies in a region approximately 5 x 5 cm in the middle of the transverse part of the trapezius muscle. Pain is radiated along the lateral upper arm and into the lateral epicondyle of humerus.

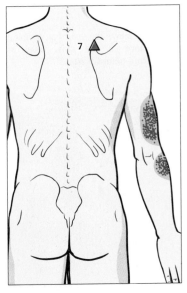

Important Acupuncture Points and Their Localizations

◉ B 10

Location: Vertical orientation: 1.3 Cun lateral to the posterior median line (Governor Vessel) in the muscle bulge of the trapezius muscle (where it just begins to descend). Acupuncture point B 10 lies 0.5 Cun cranial to the dorsal hairline, lateral to acupuncture point GV 15, close to the exit of the greater occipital nerve.
Horizontal orientation: above the spinous process of C2 (axis).

◉ B 11

Location: 1.5 Cun lateral to the lower edge of the spinous process of T1.

◉ B 12

Location: 1.5 Cun lateral to the lower edge of the spinous process of T2.

◉ GB 20

Location: In a depression between the insertions of sternocleidomastoid muscle and trapezius muscle in the region of the external occipital protuberance.

◉ GV 14

Location: Below the spinous process of C7.

◉ GV 15

Location: Above the spinous process of C2 at the same level as acupuncture point B 10, 0.5 Cun above the dorsal hairline.

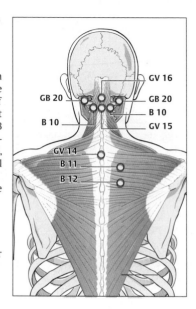

◉ GV 16

Location: Below the external occipital protuberance at the same level as acupuncture point GB 20.

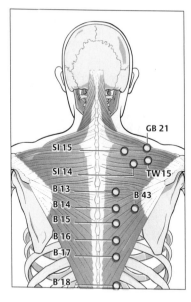

○ B 17

Location: 1.5 Cun lateral to the lower edge of the spinous process of T7.

○ B 18

Location: 1.5 Cun lateral to the lower edge of the spinous process of T9.

○ B 43

Location: 3 Cun lateral to the posterior median line, below the lower edge of the spinous process of T4.

○ SI 14

Location: 3 Cun lateral to the spinous process of T1.

○ SI 15

Location: 2 Cun lateral to the lower edge of the spinous process of C7.

○ TW 15

Location: Midway between acupuncture points GB 21 and SI 13, over the superior angle of scapula. Acupuncture point TW 15 lies approximately 1 Cun caudal to acupuncture point GB 21.

○ GB 21

Location: In the center of the connecting line between the acromion and spinous process of C7, on the dorsal elongation of mammillary line.

○ B 13

Location: 1.5 Cun lateral to the lower edge of the spinous process of T3.

○ B 14

Location: 1.5 Cun lateral to the lower edge of the spinous process of T4.

○ B 15

Location: 1.5 Cun lateral to the lower edge of the spinous process of T5.

○ B 16

Location: 1.5 Cun lateral to the lower edge of the spinous process of T6.

Gnathological Aspects of the Trapezius Muscle, Transverse Part

Functional aspects:
Bilateral activity: extends cervical spine and thoracic spine;
unilateral activity: raises, rotates and retracts the scapula;
mediotrusion in the narrower sense: masticatory muscle; stabilizes the neck during chewing.

Palpation:
Upper margin: from neck to acromion.

Symptomatology:
Occipital headache,
pain in the shoulder,
stiff shoulder,
increases all pain in the masticatory muscles, especially in the temporal muscle, masseter muscle, lateral pterygoid muscle, and sternocleidomastoid muscle.

Projected pain:
Into the neck,
occipital, in the insertion area of the splenius capitis muscle,
extends from behind the ear, across the ear, and into the temporal region,
into the submaxillary angle,
molars of lower jaws,
vertigo.

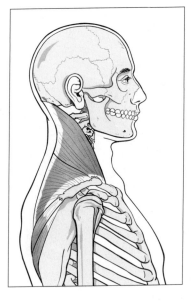

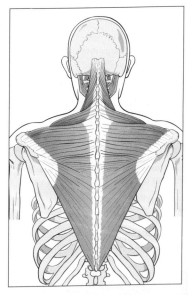

Description of the Muscle

Origin: Posterior tubercles of transverse processes of C1 to C4.

Insertion: Superior angle of scapula.

Innervation: Dorsal nerve of scapula (C3 to C5).

Action: Retracts scapula after elevation (raises supreme angle of scapula medially and cranially).

Trigger Points of the Levator Muscle of Scapula

Preliminary Remarks

The two trigger points of the levator muscle of scapula frequently cause ongoing severe discomfort. They can be activated by acute strain (e.g., long car drives) but more often by chronic shortening of the muscles through increased innervation of the postural muscles because of poor posture. Less often, the trigger points are activated in tennis players and in swimmers, or in connection with infections. Such activation is also observed in connection with the constant use of below-elbow crutches and in psychosomatic disorders.

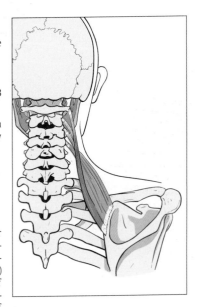

Examination of Trigger Points

The patient is examined while lying on his/her side, with the head supported in order to avoid lateral flexion of the cervical spine. The trigger points are palpated right at the insertion at the superior angle of scapula, and in the part of the muscle above the superior angle of scapula, respectively. Characteristically, prominent taut bands are palpated close to the insertion.

Therapy of Trigger Points

Deactivation through conventional acupuncture, loosening of taut bands by means of intramuscular stimulation, or alternatively trigger point infiltration. Stretching of the muscle is achieved while the patient is sitting and actively fixing the ipsilateral shoulder (e.g., on a chair) and by means of passive stretching through inclination and lateral flexion of the cervical spine using postisometric relaxation.

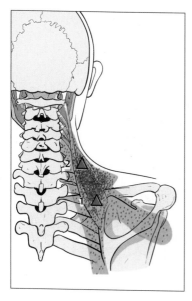

Trigger Points and Areas of Pain Projection

▲ **Levator Scapulae Muscle, Trigger Points 1 and 2**

Trigger point 1 lies close to the medial margin of the superior angle of scapula, whereas trigger point 2 lies at the transition between the transverse part and descending part of the trapezius muscle. Areas of pain projection are found around the trigger points, with radiation into the upper dorsolateral part of the deltoid muscle and along the medial margin of scapula.

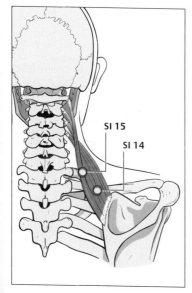

Important Acupuncture Points and Their Localizations

● **SI 14**

Location: 3 Cun lateral to the spinous process of T1.

● **SI 15**

Location: 2 Cun lateral to the lower edge of the spinous process of C7.

Gnathological Aspects of the Levator Muscle of Scapula

Functional aspects:
Elevator muscle of scapula,
rotates the neck when scapula is fixed,
responsible for the symmetry of head posture,
helps lifting and carrying heavy loads,
masticatory muscle in the narrower sense because it holds the head in a stable position when chewing; often painful in case of parafunction.

Palpation:
Medial to the cranial angle of clavicle.
Caution! Possible confusion with upper margin of trapezius muscle.

Symptomatology:
Torticollis,
pain in the shoulder at the transition to the neck,
painful "driver's neck,"
stiff neck,
stiff shoulder.

Projected pain:
Lateral into the neck,
into the superior angle of scapula.

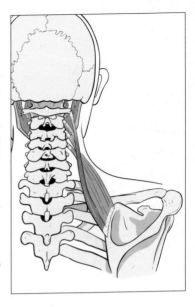

Description of the Muscle

Origin: Sternal head: upper margin of the manubrium of sternum;
clavicular head: upper margin of the medial third of clavicle.

Insertion: Mastoid process and extending toward the superior nuchal line of the occipital bone.

Innervation: Accessory nerve (11th cranial nerve).

Action: Unilateral contraction: flexes the head ipsilaterally and rotates it to the opposite side;
bilateral contraction: extends the cervical spine dorsally.

Miscellaneous: The main branches of the cervical plexus come out of the middle third of the muscle's posterior margin; at about the same level of the muscle's anterior margin lies the carotid triangle with the ramification of the common carotid artery and the first branches of the external carotid artery.

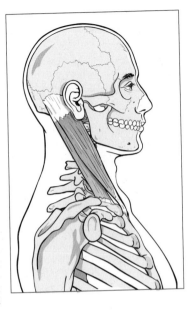

Trigger Points of the Sternocleidomastoid Muscle

Preliminary Remarks

There are seven trigger points, four of which are localized in the sternal portion of the sternocleidomastoid muscle and three in the clavicular portion. Apart from acute strain or acute reactions (e.g., after cervical whiplash injury or hangover headache after excessive alcohol consumption), the following activating factors should be considered: chronic muscular strain due to false distribution of weight (especially in connection with both scoliosis and sternosymphyseal strain position), but also chronic sinusitis or tooth infection. Rare causes are leakage after cerebrospinal fluid puncture or diskectomy. Associated trigger points are mainly localized in the contralateral sternocleidomastoid muscle, but also in all dorsal neck muscles and in the temporomandibular system. In the area of the lower trigger points of the sternal portion, arthritis of the sternoclavicular joint should be ruled out by differential diagnosis. Differential diagnosis should also consider eye, nose, and throat disorders (e.g., Ménière's disease), Horner's syndrome (cluster headache), and torticollis in a broad sense.

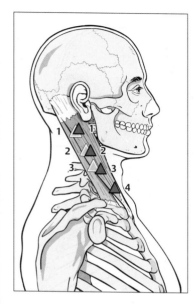

Examination of Trigger Points

While the patient is sitting and the head is fixed in neutral position, the sternal portion of the sternocleidomastoid muscle is thoroughly palpated using the forceps grip. The deeper lying portions of the clavicular part are best examined using the forceps grip while the patient is lying down and the cervical spine is flexed ipsilaterally. Again, one should distinguish between taut bands and areas of pain projection.

Therapy of Trigger Points

Conventional needling of trigger points, inactivation by means of therapeutic local anesthesia and, if necessary, dissolution of taut bands by means of intramuscular stimulation, while avoiding the underlying vascular and neural structures. Passive stretching of the clavicular part through rotation of the head toward the opposite side, moderate reclination, and simultaneous lateral flexion to the opposite side. Stretching of the sternal part is achieved through ipsilateral rotation with ipsilateral flexion. Again, it is best to use postisometric relaxation.

Trigger Points and Areas of Pain Projection

▲ Sternocleidomastoid Muscle (Sternal Part), Trigger Points 1 to 4

The four trigger points of the sternal part of the sternocleidomastoid muscle have their main projection areas in the occipital region above the mastoid process and at the level of the sternoclavicular joint. An arched area of projected pain starts at the medial side of the eyebrow and radiates in lateral direction toward the ear and the zygomatic arch. Variable areas of pain are described at the level of upper and lower jaws, in the tip of the chin, below the mandible, and in the region of the parietal bone.

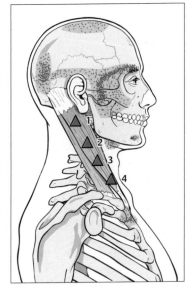

▲ Sternocleidomastoid Muscle (Clavicular Part), Trigger Points 1 to 3

The three trigger points of the clavicular part have their projection areas mainly at the level of the ear, behind the auricula and in the front above both eyes.

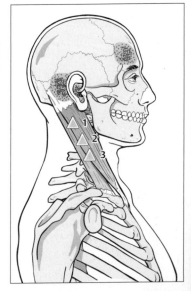

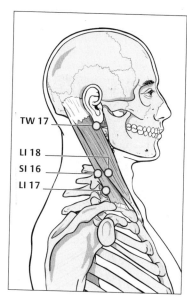

Important Acupuncture Points and Their Localizations

◯ **LI 17**

Location: 1 Cun caudal to acupuncture point LI 18, at the posterior margin of sternocleidomastoid muscle.

◯ **LI 18**

Location: At the level of the thyroid cartilage between the sternal and clavicular heads of sternocleidomastoid muscle.

◯ **SI 16**

Location: Posterior margin of sternocleidomastoid muscle, at the level of the laryngeal prominence.

◯ **TW 17**

Location: Behind the ear lobe between the lower jaw and mastoid process.

◯ **St 9**

Location: At the level of the thyroid cartilage, right in front of the sternocleidomastoid muscle. Pulsation of the carotid artery is palpable here.

◯ **St 10**

Location: Anterior margin of sternocleidomastoid muscle, in the middle of the connecting line between acupuncture points St 9 and M 11 (acupuncture point St 11: below acupuncture point St 9, at the upper margin of the clavicle, between the two heads of sternocleidomastoid muscle).

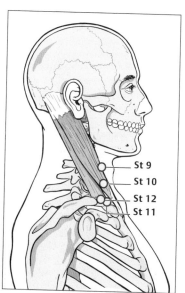

◯ **St 12**

Location: Center of the supraclavicular fossa, 4 Cun lateral to the median line as well as lateral to the clavicular part of the sternocleidomastoid muscle.

Gnathological Aspects of the Sternocleidomastoid Muscle

Functional aspects:
Bilateral activity: holds head in upright position;
unilateral activity: "dove posture"

▶ rotates the head to the opposite side,
▶ inclines the head on the same side,
▶ raises the chin (the head) on the opposite side.

Palpation:
Insertion at the mastoid process,
sternal origin, clavicular origin,
at various positions in the muscle's belly.

Symptomatology:
Faulty posture of the head toward the front,
headache of any localization (called "atypical" facial neuralgia, tension headache, and cervical cephalalgia), hemi-

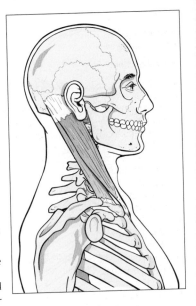

crania.

Projected pain:
No pain in the neck.

Sternal portion:

▶ into the crown of the head;
▶ into the occiput;
▶ into the eye, around the eye and deep behind the eye (often with lacrimation, reddened conjunctiva, drooping of the upper eyelid, impaired vision);
▶ two-dimensionally into the lateral face (then often erroneously called "atypical" facial neuralgia);
▶ across the cheek;
▶ into the lateral upper jaw;
▶ into the acoustic meatus;
▶ into the region of the hyoid bone and larynx;
▶ difficulty in swallowing and sensation of a soar throat;
▶ into the sternum;
▶ into a small spot lateral to the chin;
▶ sometimes ringing in the ears or even tinnitus.

Clavicular portion:

▶ toward the front: frontal headache;
▶ in the front, often also from the ipsilateral direction;
▶ projecting in contralateral direction and into the ear (often confused with otitis media).

Retroauricular portion:

▶ into the cheek;
▶ diffuse into the teeth of the lateral upper jaw;
▶ feeling dizzy with imaginary movements and sensations in the head, rarely vertigo;
▶ disturbed balance.

Description of the Muscle

Origin: Clavicular head: medial half of clavicle;
sternocostal head: anterior plane of sternum and costal cartilages of the six upper ribs;
abdominal part: anterior plate of the rectus sheath.

Insertion: Crest of lesser tubercle of humerus (the lower parts insert most cranially).

Innervation: Medial and lateral pectoral nerves (C5 to T1).

Action: Adducts, flexes, and rotates the arm inwards, lowers the shoulder, retracts scapula after elevation, accessory respiratory muscle.

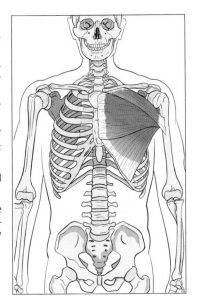

Trigger Points of the Greater Pectoral Muscle

Preliminary Remarks

This muscle has trigger points in five different areas according to its anatomical structure. Active trigger points can be expected to be common in case of sternosymphyseal strain position (with shoulders rotated to the front), but also in case of acute strain (carrying heavy items) or in case of unaccustomed physical stress. However, symptoms with projection to the upper anterior thoracic region also appear in cases of symptomatic coronary heart disease and heart attack. Persistent symptoms following such an event, on the other hand, point to active trigger points of the greater pectoral muscle.

Examination of Trigger Points

Local twitch responses can often be triggered by direct palpation or by using the forceps grip at the lateral part of the muscle while the muscle is stretched in a targeted way by horizontal abduction of the arm and simultaneous retraction of the shoulder joints.

Therapy of Trigger Points

By conventional needling or, alternatively, therapeutic local anesthesia and by targeted dissolution of taut bands using intramuscular stimulation. This is followed by passive stretching of the muscle with the arm rotated outwards and the shoulders retracted.

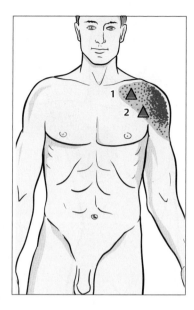

Trigger Points and Areas of Pain Projection

▲ **Greater Pectoral Muscle (Clavicular Head of the Left Greater Pectoral Muscle), Trigger Points 1 and 2**

There are two trigger points in the middle third of the clavicular head; their main areas of projection lie at the ventral portion of the deltoid muscle. This applies only to the left greater pectoral muscle.

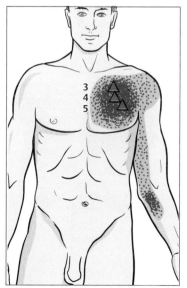

▲ **Greater Pectoral Muscle (Sternocostal Head of the Left Greater Pectoral Muscle), Trigger Points 3 to 5**

The three trigger points of the sternocostal part have their main projection areas directly over the greater pectoral muscle. Another projection area is found close to the origin at the level of the flexor muscle of the ulnar carpus and on the inside of the upper arm as well as close to the middle and ring fingers. This applies only to the left greater pectoral muscle.

▲ **Greater Pectoral Muscle (Abdominal Part of the Left Greater Pectoral Muscle), Trigger Points 6 and 7**

The two trigger points of the abdominal part lie right in front of the muscle's entrance into the axillary fossa. Their main projection areas are found medial and distant to the trigger points at the level of the mammilla. This applies only to the left greater pectoral muscle.

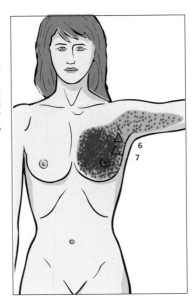

▲ **Greater Pectoral Muscle (Sternocostal Head of the Right Greater Pectoral Muscle), Trigger Points 1 and 2**

These two trigger points are localized close to the sternum in the sternocostal part of the greater pectoral muscle and have their main areas of pain projection in this region. This applies only to the right greater pectoral muscle.

▲ **Greater Pectoral Muscle (Abdominal Part of the Right Greater Pectoral Muscle), Trigger Point 3**

Another trigger point is localized in the middle of the abdominal part of the muscle and shows a correlation with arrhythmic heart beat. This applies only to the right greater pectoral muscle.

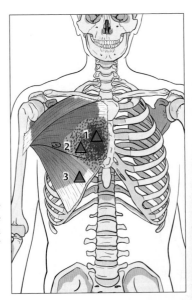

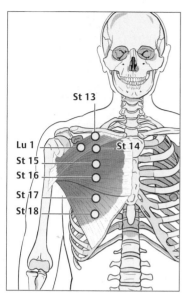

Important Acupuncture Points and Their Localizations

○ Lu 1

Location: 6 Cun lateral to the anterior median line, 1 Cun below the clavicle, slightly medial to the caudal border of the coracoid process at the level of the first intercostal space (ICS 1).

○ St 13

Location: At the lower edge of the clavicle, 4 Cun lateral to the anterior median line.

○ St 14

Location: Within ICS 1 on the mammillary line, 4 Cun lateral to the anterior median line.

○ St 15

Location: Within ICS 2 on the mammillary line, 4 Cun lateral to the anterior median line.

○ St 16

Location: Within ICS 3 on the mammillary line, 4 Cun lateral to the anterior median line.

○ St 17

Location: Within ICS 4 at the mammilla, 4 Cun lateral to the anterior median line.

○ St 18

Location: Within ICS 5 on the mammillary line, 4 Cun lateral to the anterior median line.

○ **Sp 18**

Location: Within ICS 4, 2 Cun lateral and slightly cranial to the mammilla. (Note the ascending aspect of the intercostal space.)

○ **Sp 19**

Location: Within ICS 3, 2 Cun lateral to the mammillary line.

○ **Sp 20**

Location: Within ICS 2, 2 Cun lateral to the cranially extended mammillary line.

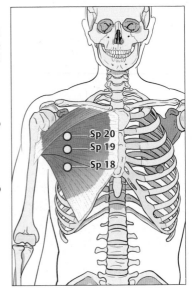

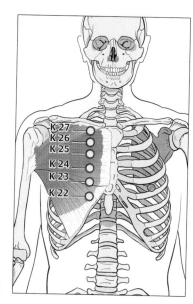

○ **K 22**

Location: Within ICS 5, 2 Cun lateral to the anterior median line.

○ **K 23**

Location: Within ICS 4, 2 Cun lateral to the anterior median line.

○ **K 24**

Location: Within ICS 3, 2 Cun lateral to the anterior median line.

○ **K 25**

Location: Within ICS 2, 2 Cun lateral to the anterior median line.

○ **K 26**

Location: Within ICS 1, 2 Cun lateral to the anterior median line.

○ **K 27**

Location: Right under the clavicle, 2 Cun lateral to the anterior median line.

Description of the Muscle

Origin: End of bony portions of the 3rd to 5th rib.

Insertion: Coracoid process of scapula with a short, flat tendon (together with tendon of the coracobrachial muscle and short head of the biceps brachii muscle).

Innervation: Medial (C8/T1) and lateral (C5 to C7) pectoral nerves.

Action: Lowers the scapula; raises the ribs when the arm is fixed (accessory respiratory muscle).

Trigger Points of the Smaller Pectoral Muscle

Preliminary Remarks

This muscle tends to become shorter. Clinically, neurovascular disturbances of the thoracic outlet syndrome are very much in evidence, especially when the arm is rotated outwards and abducted more than 140°, due to physiological tightness caused by compression of the brachial artery and brachial nerve trunks. Two trigger point localizations are known; however, they often appear in combination with trigger points of the greater pectoral muscle and subclavius muscle.

Examination of Trigger Points

While the patient is lying on his/her back with the arm abducted approximately 80° and rotated outwards, the trigger points can be directly palpated. The trigger point close to the origin at the level of the 4th rib is palpated under the greater pectoral muscle with either the index finger or thumb after gripping the greater pectoral muscle using the forceps grip.

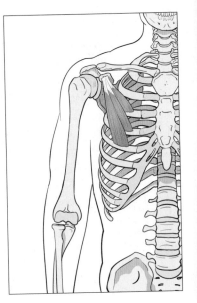

Therapy of Trigger Points

In the position described for examination, the trigger points can be either needled directly or inactivated by dry-needling or therapeutic local anesthesia. In case of the trigger point close to the insertion, one should consider the risk of damaging the neurovascular structures underlying the tendon. Treatment is completed by passive stretching of the muscle through abduction, external rotation, and retroversion of the arm using postisometric relaxation.

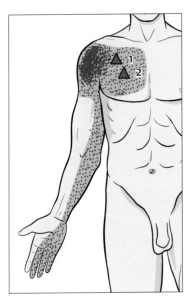

Trigger Points and Areas of Pain Projection

▲ Smaller Pectoral Muscle, Trigger Points 1 and 2

There is only one area of pain projection for both trigger points; it is predominantly localized over the anterior portion of the shoulder joint. The pain radiates across the thoracic muscles and along the entire ulnar side of the upper and lower arm, radiating into the middle to little fingers. One trigger point is located close to the origin at the level of the 4th rib, the other one close to the insertion approximately 1 to 2 Cun caudal to the coracoid process.

Important Acupuncture Points and Their Localizations

● Lu 1

Location: At the level of ICS 1, 6 Cun lateral to the anterior median line, 1 Cun below the clavicle, slightly medial to the caudal border of the coracoid process.

● St 15

Location: Within ICS 2 on the mammillary line, 4 Cun lateral to the anterior median line.

● St 16

Location: Within ICS 3 on the mammillary line, 4 Cun lateral to the anterior median line.

● St 17

Location: Within ICS 4 at the mammilla, 4 Cun lateral to the anterior median line.

● Sp 19

Location: Within ICS 3, 2 Cun lateral to the mammillary line.

● Sp 20

Location: Within ICS 2, 2 Cun lateral to the cranially extended mammillary line.

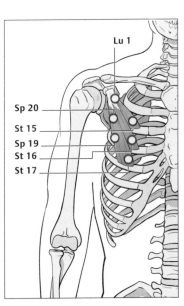

Description of the Muscles

Smaller Rhomboid Muscle

Origin: Spinous processes of C6 and C7.

Insertion: Upper medial margin of scapula.

Innervation: Dorsal nerve of scapula (C4/C5).

Action: Retracts scapula after elevation.

Greater Rhomboid Muscle

Origin: Spinous processes of T1 to T4.

Insertion: Medial margin of scapula.

Innervation: Dorsal nerve of scapula (C4/C5).

Action: Retracts scapula after elevation.

Trigger Points of Smaller and Greater Rhomboid Muscles

Preliminary Remarks

There are two trigger points in the greater rhomboid muscle and one trigger point in the smaller rhomboid muscle. Activation of the trigger points is found mainly after strain, especially caused by the sternosymphyseal strain position with round back. Associated trigger points can be found in the levator muscle of scapula, the infraspinatus muscle, and the central portion of the trapezius muscle.

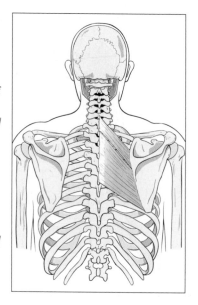

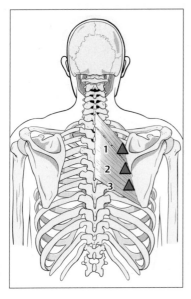

Examination of Trigger Points

While the patient is sitting in the round-back position, the trigger points can be easily identified at the medial margin of the scapula.

Therapy of Trigger Points

Inactivation of these trigger points is rapidly achieved by means of dry-needling, conventional acupuncture, or therapeutic local anesthesia using the tangential puncture technique to avoid pneumothorax.

Trigger Points and Areas of Pain Projection

▲ **Smaller and Greater Rhomboid Muscles, Trigger Points 1 to 3**

The trigger point in the smaller rhomboid muscle is approximately 3 cm medial to the medial margin of the scapula. The two trigger points of the greater rhomboid muscle are localized more caudally, again approximately 3 cm medial to the medial margin of the scapula. The areas of pain projection of all three trigger points are found around the medial margin of the scapula and the supraspinous fossa.

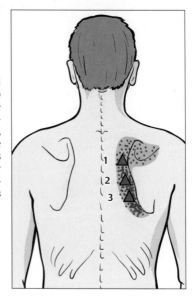

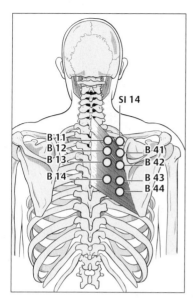

Important Acupuncture Points and Their Localizations

◯ **SI 14**

Location: 3 Cun lateral to the lower edge of the spinous process of T1.

◯ **B 11**

Location: 1.5 Cun lateral to the lower edge of the spinous process of T1.

◯ **B 12**

Location: 1.5 Cun lateral to the lower edge of the spinous process of T2.

◯ **B 13**

Location: 1.5 Cun lateral to the lower edge of the spinous process of T3.

◯ **B 14**

Location: 1.5 Cun lateral to the lower edge of the spinous process of T4.

◯ **B 41**

Location: 3 Cun lateral to the lower edge of the spinous process of T2.

◯ **B 42**

Location: 3 Cun lateral to the lower edge of the spinous process of T3.

◯ **B 43**

Location: 3 Cun lateral to the lower edge of the spinous process of T4.

◯ **B 44**

Location: 3 Cun lateral to the lower edge of the spinous process of T5.

Description of the Muscle

Origin: Supraspinous fossa of scapula.

Insertion: Upper edge of the greater tubercle of humerus, extending into the joint capsule (muscle of rotator cuff).

Innervation: Suprascapular nerve (C4 to C6).

Action: Abducts humerus; tightens the joint capsule.

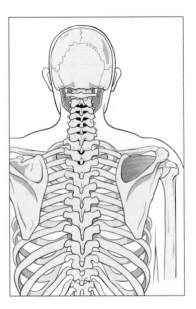

Trigger Points of the Supraspinatus Muscle

Preliminary Remarks

There are three trigger points, two of them in the muscle belly and one in the region of the supraspinous tendon. Activation of the trigger points occurs mostly in situations of acute strain (e.g., carrying heavy loads without being used to it), but also in chronic overloading syndromes. The trigger points are usually associated with those in the trapezius muscle, infraspinatus muscle and latissimus dorsi muscle.

Examination of Trigger Points

While the patient is sitting, the trigger points are directly palpated in the muscle belly and close to the insertion, triggering a typical referred pain.

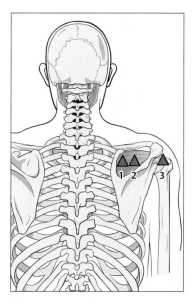

Therapy of Trigger Points

Inactivation of the trigger points is usually achieved without any problem by means of acupuncture, therapeutic local anesthesia, or dry-needling. When injecting into the trigger point of the supraspinous tendon, meticulously sterile conditions should be observed because of the vicinity of the joint. The muscle is stretched by adducting and maximally rotating the upper arm inwards, while simultaneously rotating the arm slightly to the back.

Trigger Points and Areas of Pain Projection

▲ Supraspinatus Muscle, Trigger Points 1 and 2

The trigger points lie in the muscle belly, one at the transition of the acromion to the spine of scapula, and the other one in the infraspinous fossa close to the origin and the medial margin of the scapula. Patients complain about radiating pain with the main projection area over the deltoid muscle and also over the head of radius, and about minor pain radiating into the region of the dorsal shoulder girdle, the dorsolateral and ventral upper and lower arm.

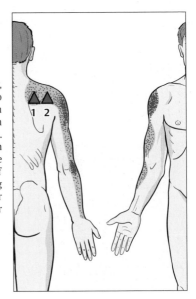

▲ Supraspinatus Muscle, Trigger Point 3

The trigger point in the supraspinous tendon has its main projection area over the deltoid muscle.

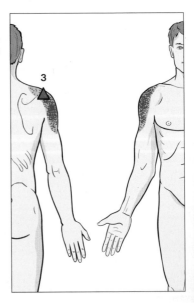

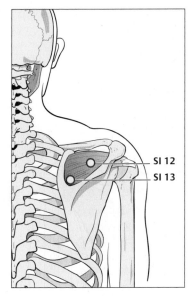

Important Acupuncture Points and Their Localizations

⬤ SI 12

Location: Approximately 1 Cun above the middle of the cranial border of the spine of scapula, cranial to acupoint SI 11.

⬤ SI 13

Location: Right above the spine of scapula, in the middle of the connecting line between acupoint SI 10 and the spinous process (lower pole) of T2.

Description of the Muscle

Origin: Infraspinous fossa of scapula.

Insertion: Middle and lower third of the greater tubercle of humerus, joint capsule.

Innervation: Suprascapular nerve (C4 to C6).

Action: Rotates arm outwards;
upper part: abduction,
lower part: adduction.

Miscellaneous: The infraspinatus muscle belongs to the muscles of the rotator cuff because it extends into the capsule of the shoulder joint.

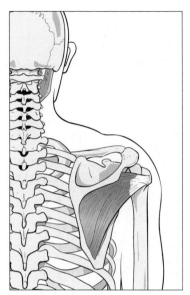

Trigger Points of the Infraspinatus Muscle

Preliminary Remarks

Two trigger points are found predominantly; a third trigger point appears variably at the medial margin at the level of the middle of the infraspinous fossa. The trigger points are activated by unaccustomed sports activities (e.g., excessive playing of tennis). Differential diagnosis should consider structural disorders of the shoulder joint, stiffness of the shoulder, and affection of the nerve roots C5, C6, and C7.

Examination of Trigger Points

Provocation is achieved by abducting the arm and maximally rotating it inwards in the shoulder joint to stretch the infraspinatus muscle. When the arms are relaxed, typical taut bands are found caudal to the spine of scapula.

Therapy of Trigger Points

Targeted needling of trigger points and dissolving the muscular shortening by means of dry-needling. Therapeutic local anesthesia is also possible. This is followed by passive stretching of the muscles through retroversion and internal rotation of the arm.

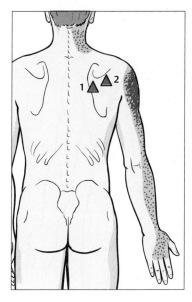

Trigger Points and Areas of Pain Projection

▲ **Infraspinatus Muscle, Trigger Points 1 and 2**

Both trigger points are localized in the medial half of the muscle, approximately 2 Cun below the scapular spine. There are areas of pain projection over the dorsal as well as ventral portion of the deltoid muscle with radiation into the dorsal and ventral upper and lower arm on the radial side.

Trigger Points and Areas of Pain Projection

▲ **Infraspinatus Muscle, Trigger Point 3**

A third trigger point lies at the medio-caudal origin and has its main area of pain projection at the medial margin of scapula. It appears only occasionally.

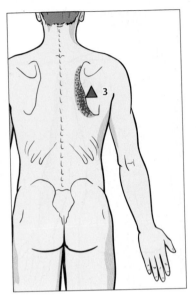

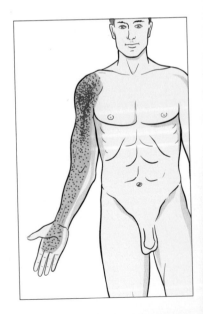

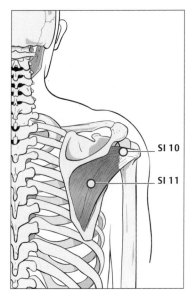

Important Acupuncture Points and Their Localizations

○ **SI 10**

Location: Right above acupoint SI 9, below the well palpable scapular spine.

○ **SI 11**

Location: In the infraspinous fossa on the connecting line between the middle of the well palpable scapular spine and the inferior angle of scapula. Acupoint SI 11 lies between the cranial third and the other two-thirds of this line.

Description of the Muscle

Origin: Subscapular fossa of scapula (not at the neck of scapula)

Insertion: Lesser tubercle of humerus and proximal crest of lesser tubercle.

Innervation: Subscapular nerve (C5/C6).

Action: Rotates the arm inwards; tightens the joint capsule into which the subscapular muscle extends as well (muscle of the rotator cuff).

Trigger Points of the Subscapular Muscle

Preliminary Remarks

There are three trigger points here; because of the location of the muscle, however, they are difficult to get at for treatment. Trigger points of this muscle appear usually as a result of chronic changes, which are generally summarized under the term "frozen shoulder." The trigger points of the subscapular muscle appear usually in combination with those of the following muscles: greater pectoral muscle, teres major muscle, latissimus dorsi muscle, and the long head of triceps muscle.

Examination of Trigger Points

With the patient lying on his/her back and under slight traction of the arm with approximately 90° abduction and internal rotation, the anterior side of the scapula is palpated medially to the latissimus dorsi muscle using the thumb of the other hand. Local twitch responses can be triggered in the region of the activated trigger points.

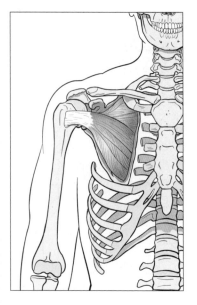

Therapy of Trigger Points

Targeted needling, dry-needling, and therapeutic local anesthesia may be applied. However, distinctly longer needles and injection needles are required (approx. 7 to 8 cm in length). Treatment is followed by stretching the muscle by external rotation and up to 90° abduction; the latter can be successively increased to up to 180°. These physiotherapeutic methods are supported by postisometric relaxation.

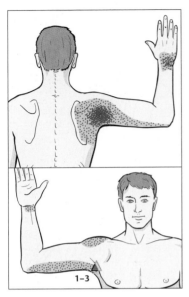

Trigger Points and Areas of Pain Projection

▲ **Subscapular Muscle, Trigger Points 1 to 3**

The three trigger points can be found in the cranial and central thirds of the muscle. Their common areas of pain projection present at the dorsal upper arm, including the scapula, over the deltoid muscle as well as the dorsal and ventral aspects of the wrist.

Important Acupuncture Points and Their Localizations

The muscle is anatomically inaccessible for direct acupuncture.

Description of the Muscle

Origin: Lateral supraepicondylar ridge of humerus.

Insertion: Base of metacarpal bone II.

Innervation: Deep branch of radial nerve (C6/C7).

Action: Extends and radially abducts the wrist.

Trigger Points of the Long Radial Extensor Muscle of Wrist

Preliminary Remarks

There is one main trigger point zone here. Trigger points in this region are common. Activation usually occurs due to muscular imbalance between the extensor and flexor muscles of the lower arm. Associated trigger points are found in the extensor muscle of fingers, supinator muscle, and brachioradial muscle.

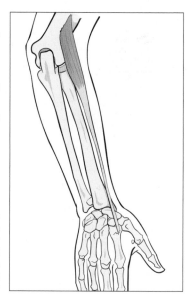

Examination of Trigger Points

With the wrist slightly flexed and the fingers flexed, vigorous local twitch responses can be triggered quite frequently by direct palpation of the respective muscle. Trigger points can also be quickly diagnosed by isometric testing.

Therapy of Trigger Points

Extremely successful are, on the one hand, conventional acupuncture and therapeutic local anesthesia and, on the other hand, targeted intramuscular stimulation by means of acupuncture needles. Passive stretching of the muscles—supported by postisometric relaxation, if necessary—will prevent relapses.

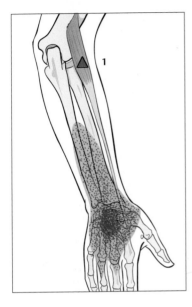

Trigger Points and Areas of Pain Projection

▲ Long Radial Extensor Muscle of Wrist, Trigger Point 1

This trigger point lies in the muscle belly at the level of the head of the radius. Its areas of pain projection lie over the head of the radius and dorsal to that over the abductor muscle of thumb.

Important Acupuncture Points and Their Localizations

○ LI 8

Location: On the connecting line between acupoints LI 5 and LI 11, two-thirds proximal to acupoint LI 5 and one third distal to acupoint LI 11; hence, acupoint LI 8 lies 4 Cun distal to LI 11.

○ LI 9

Location: 3 Cun distal to acupoint LI 11.

○ LI 10

Location: 2 Cun distal to acupoint LI 11. LI 11

Location: Lateral to the radial end of the flexion crease of the elbow when the lower arm is flexed at a right angle, in a depression between the end of the crease and the lateral epicondyle in the region of the long radial extensor muscle of the wrist.

○ LI 12

Location: 1 Cun obliquely above acupoint LI 11, close to the humerus.

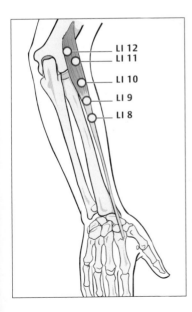

Description of the Muscle

Origin: Lateral epicondyle of humerus, annular and collateral ligaments of radius, fascia of lower arm.

Insertion: Dorsal aponeurosis; proximal to the middle finger joints, the aponeurosis divides into the ulnar and radial tendinous portions that reunite distally to the joint in an aponeurosis and insert at the base of the terminal phalanges.

Innervation: Deep branch of radial nerve (C6 to C8).

Action: Extends finger joints, extends wrist, and supports ulnar abduction.

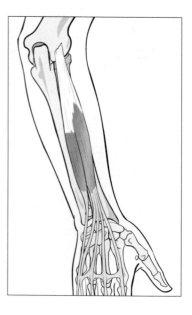

Trigger Points of the Extensor Muscle of Fingers

Preliminary Remarks

Trigger points are found here predominantly in the muscle bellies of the extensor muscles of the ring and middle fingers. Activation of trigger points usually takes place through chronic strain. Associated trigger points are often also present in the finger muscles and the extensor muscle of wrist.

Examination of Trigger Points

Typical local twitch responses can be triggered in the middle of the muscle belly in the region of the trigger points.

Therapy of Trigger Points

Targeted intramuscular stimulation with subsequent passive stretching of the muscle is effective within a short time. Conventional needling and therapeutic local anesthesia may also be considered.

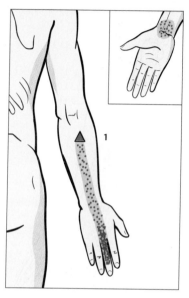

Trigger Points and Areas of Pain Projection

▲ Extensor Muscle of Fingers, Trigger Point 1

The trigger point of the middle finger extensor is found close to the elbow in the region of the muscle belly. Typical pain projection runs along the muscle into the middle finger; now and then pain is also localized over the proximal flexion crease of the wrist.

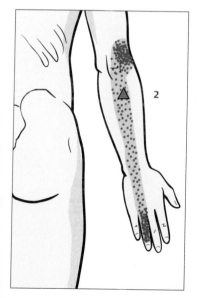

▲ Extensor Muscle of Fingers, Trigger Point 2

The trigger point of the ring finger extensor lies distal and ulnar to trigger point 1. Its area of pain projection reaches into the ring finger and up toward the radiohumeral joint.

Important Acupuncture Points and Their Localizations

◉ **LI 8**

Location: 4 Cun distal to acupoint LI 11.

◉ **LI 9**

Location: 3 Cun distal to acupoint LI 11.

◉ **LI 10**

Location: 2 Cun distal to acupoint LI 11.

◉ **LI 11**

Location: Lateral to the radial end of the flexion crease of elbow when the lower arm is flexed at a right angle, in a depression between the end of the crease and the lateral epicondyle in the region of the long radial extensor of the wrist.

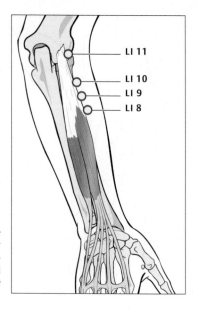

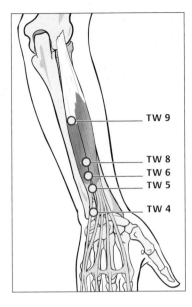

TW 9

TW 8
TW 6
TW 5

TW 4

○ TW 4

Location: Slightly ulnar to the center of the dorsal flexion crease of the wrist (the joint space between radius, ulna, and proximal wrist bone series), ulnar to the tendon of the extensor muscle of fingers, radial to the tendon of the extensor muscle of little finger.

○ TW 5

Location: 2 Cun proximal to acupoint TW 4, between the radius and ulna, on a line connecting acupoint TW 4 and the tip of the olecranon process of ulna.

○ TW 6

Location: 3 Cun proximal to acupoint TW 4, between the radius and ulna, on the line connecting acupoint TW 4 and the tip of the olecranon.

○ TW 8

Location: 4 Cun proximal to acupoint TW 4, between the radius and ulna.

○ TW 9

Location: 7 Cun proximal to acupoint TW 4 on the line connecting acupoint TW 4 and the tip of the olecranon. Hence, on the connecting line described, the point lies 1 Cun proximal to the middle between acupoint TW 4 and the flexion crease of elbow.

Description of the Muscle

Origin of the iliacus muscle: The iliac fossa up to the terminal line of pelvis, anterior inferior iliac spine, lacuna of muscles up to the anterior surface of the hip joint capsule.

Origin of the greater psoas muscle: Superficially from the sides of vertebrae T12 and L1 to L4 and also the associated disks; deep layer from the costal processes of the lumbar vertebrae.

Common insertion: As iliopsoas muscle at the lesser trochanter of femur.

Innervation: Femoral nerve (T12 to L3 [L4]).

Action: The strongest flexor muscle of the hip joint: bends the lumbar spine (at the fixed point on the femur); unilateral contraction of the greater psoas muscle bends the lumbar spine laterally.

Miscellaneous: Between the two portions of the greater psoas muscle lies the lumbar plexus.

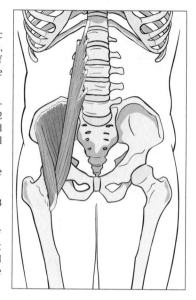

Trigger Points of the Iliopsoas Muscle

Preliminary Remarks

This muscle is divided into the smaller psoas muscle, greater psoas muscle, and iliacus muscle. Three trigger points are found here. Trigger points in this region are very common because of the muscle's general tendency to shorten. This can usually be observed in chronic overloading syndromes and improper strains of the muscle, which become manifest as lumbar spine syndrome and also as coxarthrosis. The trigger points normally appear in combination with those in other muscles (e.g., quadratus lumborum muscle, straight abdominal muscle, rectus femoris muscle, and tensor muscle of fascia lata), but also in the contralateral iliopsoas muscle. In each case, treatment of the associated trigger points is required.

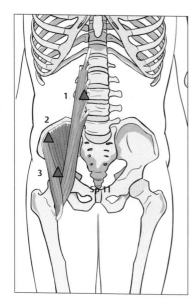

Examination of Trigger Points

The trigger points are often not directly accessible to the palpating finger. The trigger point located in the greater psoas muscle (trigger point 1) is now and then pressure sensitive on deep palpation in the relaxed patient; jump signs are absent. On the inside of the ilium, in the more anterior portion, another trigger point is found (trigger point 2), which is also only palpable in the relaxed patient lying on his/her back. An additional trigger point (trigger point 3) is found right at the level of the hip joint.

Therapy of Trigger Points

Only the distal trigger point (trigger point 3) is accessible to acupuncture and injection therapy; it is less accessible to dry-needling. The main focus of treatment is on physiotherapeutic stretching by extending the respective hip joint with maximal flexion of the contralateral hip joint. At the same time, stretching of the usually also shortened rectus femoris muscle is required.

Trigger Points and Areas of Pain Projection

▲ **Iliopsoas Muscle, Trigger Points 1 to 3**

Trigger points 1 and 2 lie in the ventral portion of the iliopsoas muscle and prevertebrally at the level of vertebra L3. Trigger point 3 lies directly above the hip joint. Their areas of pain projection are found directly paravertebrally in the lumbar region with radiation into the sacroiliac joint and the upper medial gluteal area. Another area of pain projection appears over the rectus femoris muscle with radiation toward the anterior inferior iliac spine.

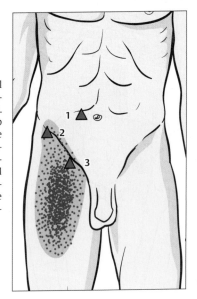

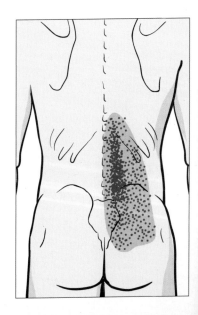

Important Acupuncture Points and Their Localizations

The muscle is anatomically inaccessible to acupuncture.

Description of the Muscle

Origin: Dorsal fibers: iliac crest and iliolumbar ligament;
ventral parts: costal processes of vertebrae L2 to L5.

Insertion: Dorsal part: 12th rib and costal processes of vertebrae L1 to L3;
ventral part: 12th rib.

Innervation: Subcostal nerve and lumbar plexus (T12 to L3).

Action: Flexes the trunk laterally, stabilizes the 12th rib during respiration (fixed point for the diaphragm).

Trigger Points of the Quadratus Lumborum Muscle

Preliminary Remarks

There are two trigger points in both the deep and superficial portions of the muscle. Disorders of the sacroiliac joint frequently present clinically. Activation of trigger points results from acute strain, also in connection with accidents, and becomes chronic in functional scoliosis (as a result of unequal lengths of the legs) or in primary scoliosis. Associated trigger points appear in the region of abdominal muscles, in the contralateral quadratus lumborum muscle, in the ipsilateral iliopsoas muscle and iliocostal muscle, and occasionally also in the latissimus dorsi muscle and internal oblique muscle of abdomen. Additional trigger points are found in the gluteal region, especially in case of symptoms of nerve root stimulation related to nerve roots L5 and S1.

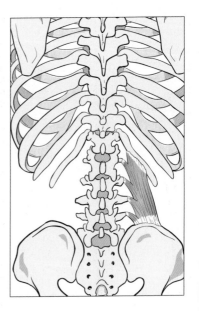

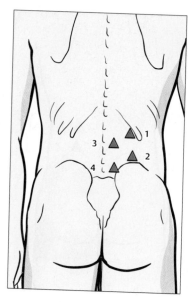

Examination of Trigger Points

First of all, the following orthopedic causes should be clarified: functional or structural scoliosis, scoliotic pelvis, oblique position of pelvis, and displacement of pelvis. Palpation of trigger points is performed while the patient is lying relaxed on his/her side. Local twitch responses are rarely observed; usually there is distinct hardening of the muscle.

Therapy of Trigger Points

Direct needling is only possible with acupuncture needles of at least 60 mm in length. Therapeutic local anesthesia is a possible alternative. However, dry-needling can usually be successfully performed as well; in lateral position, the needle is aimed in the direction of the transverse processes. As follow-up treatment, stretching the muscles is carried out in the dorsal position with the hip joint flexed approximately 80° using postisometric relaxation by adduction of the hip joint. This also stretches the entire gluteal region.

Trigger Points and Areas of Pain Projection

▲ Quadratus Lumborum Muscle, Trigger Points 1 and 2

The superficial trigger point 1 lies approximately 2 Cun below the lateral end of the muscle border and 2 Cun below the 12th rib; it shows an area of pain projection at the level of the lateral and dorsal proximal gluteal regions with radiation toward the groin and the sacroiliac joint. Trigger point 2 is found at the level of L4, just above the insertion of the quadratus lumborum muscle at the dorsolateral iliac crest. Its pain projection lies at the level of the greater trochanter and radiates in ventral and dorsal directions.

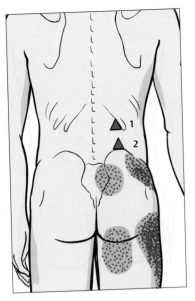

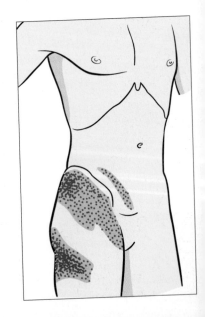

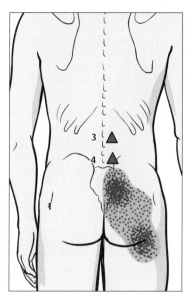

▲ Quadratus Lumborum Muscle, Trigger Points 3 and 4

Trigger points of the muscle's deep portion are localized at the level of L3 and L4; their typical projection areas are found over the sacroiliac joint and in the lower middle of the buttock.

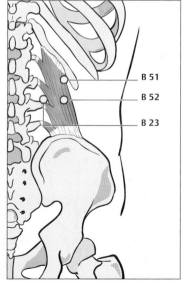

Important Acupuncture Points and Their Localizations

◉ B 23

Location: 1.5 Cun lateral to the lower edge of the spinous process of vertebra L2.

◉ B 51

Location: 3 Cun lateral to the lower edge of the spinous process of vertebra L1.

◉ B 52

Location: 3 Cun lateral to the lower edge of the spinous process of vertebra L2.

Description of the Muscle

Origin: Rectus femoris muscle: with one head at the anterior inferior iliac spine, the other at the acetabulum and hip joint capsule.
Vastus medialis muscle: distal part of the intertrochanteric line, medial lip of linea aspera.
Vastus lateralis muscle: lateral part of greater trochanter, lateral lip of linea aspera, intertrochanteric line.
Vastus intermedius muscle: anterior and lateral surfaces of femur.

Insertion: Base and lateral surface of the patella and tuberosity of tibia via the patellar ligament.

Innervation: Femoral nerve (L2 to L4); indicator muscle for L4.

Action: Extends the leg; rectus femoris muscle: flexes the thigh.

Trigger Points of the Quadriceps Fermoris Muscle

Preliminary Remarks

Trigger points in this group of muscles are very common, the symptoms being mainly restricted to the thigh; most trigger points are observed in the vastus lateralis muscle. These trigger points are activated by acute strain during sports activities, especially in the case of sudden vehement eccentric contraction. Trigger points in the quadriceps femoris muscle usually appear as a consequence of primary trigger points in the region of the dorsal thigh muscles and soleus muscle. However, primary trigger points can also be found as a result of muscular imbalance between the vastus medialis muscle and the vastus lateralis muscle when hip and knee joints are affected.

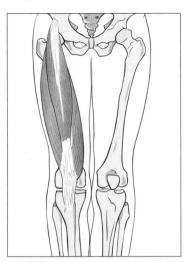

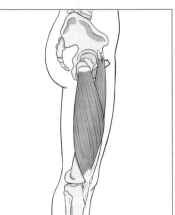

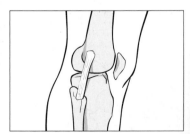

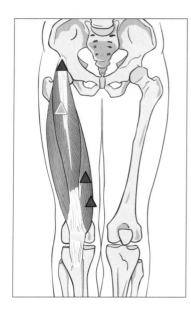

Examination of Trigger Points

With the hip joint slightly abducted, the rectus femoris muscle is examined by palpating the proximal part with the thumb. The vastus medialis muscle is grasped by direct palpation while the knee is flexed and the hip slightly flexed and abducted. At the same time, the knee joint should be supported laterally to avoid the patient actively holding the leg. The vastus intermedius muscle is palpated deep while the patient lies in the dorsal position with the leg extended and the hip and knee joints in neutral positions. Trigger points in the vastus lateralis muscle are identified once again by direct palpation with the hip and knee joints slightly flexed and the knee joint supported from below.

Therapy of Trigger Points

Dry-needling seems to be the best procedure here; typically, this triggers local twitch responses of taut bands. Consideration should also be given to acupuncture or trigger point infiltration. The patient has to be instructed to stretch the muscles adequately after treatment as they are often shortened; additional postisometric relaxation exercises are helpful.

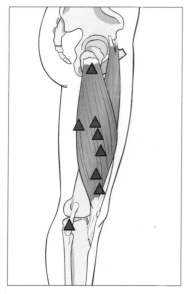

Trigger Points and Areas of Pain Projection

▲ Quadriceps Femoris Muscle (Rectus Femoris Muscle), Trigger Point 1

The trigger point of the rectus femoris muscle is localized close to the origin of the muscle, right over the hip joint. It has a typical projection area over the distal anterior thigh.

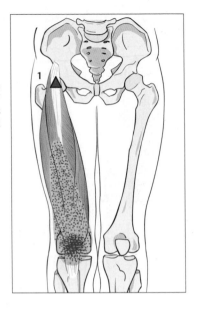

▲ Quadriceps Femoris Muscle (Vastus Intermedius Muscle), Trigger Point 1

The vastus intermedius muscle, which lies under the rectus femoris muscle, possesses trigger points in all parts of the muscle. Their appearance varies, and they lead to local radiation in the anterior thigh.

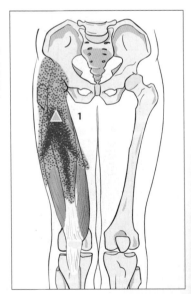

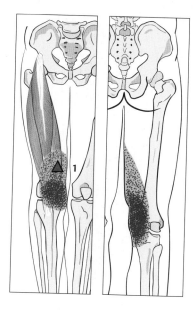

▲ **Quadriceps Femoris Muscle (Vastus Medialis Muscle), Trigger Point 1**

Trigger point 1 of the vastus medialis muscle is found in the muscle belly, 5 cm proximal to the upper pole of the patella, and leads to radiation symptoms over the medial joint space of the knee and over the distal medial thigh.

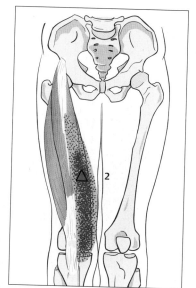

▲ **Quadriceps Femoris Muscle (Vastus Medialis Muscle), Trigger Point 2**

Trigger point 2 of the vastus medialis muscle lies in the middle of the muscle and its area of pain projection runs along the muscle, predominantly in distal direction.

▲ Quadriceps Femoris Muscle (Vastus Lateralis Muscle), Trigger Point 1

Trigger point 1 of the vastus lateralis muscle is found in the ventral part just above the patella. Its main area of pain projection lies laterally around the patella toward the lateral joint space and radiates slightly into the lateral middle portion of the thigh.

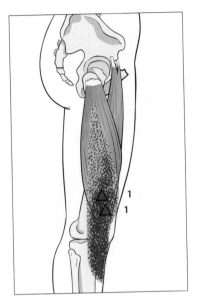

▲ Quadriceps Femoris Muscle (Vastus Lateralis Muscle), Trigger Point 2

Trigger point 2 lies just dorsal to trigger point 1. It radiates into the distal portion of the vastus lateralis muscle with further projection zones in the dorsolateral thigh and proximal dorsolateral lower leg.

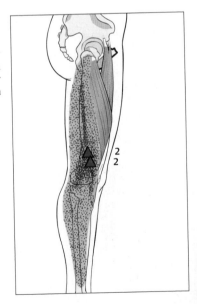

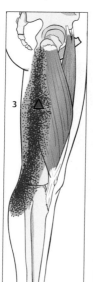
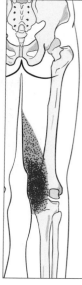

▲ Quadriceps Femoris Muscle (Vastus Lateralis Muscle), Trigger Point 3

Trigger point 3 is found in the middle of the muscle belly close to its dorsal margin; its area of pain projection reaches from the greater trochanter to the head of the fibula.

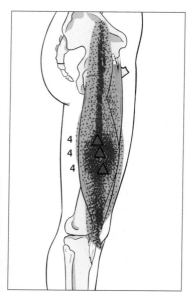

▲ Quadriceps Femoris Muscle (Vastus Lateralis Muscle), Trigger Point 4

Trigger point 4 lies exactly in the middle of the muscle belly. It leads to radiating symptoms along the femur up to the lateral gluteal region and the anterolateral knee joint region, while the patella remains free of pain.

▲ Quadriceps Femoris Muscle (Vastus Lateralis Muscle), Trigger Point 5

Trigger point 5 is found right below the greater trochanter at the origin of the muscle, and here is its local area of pain radiation.

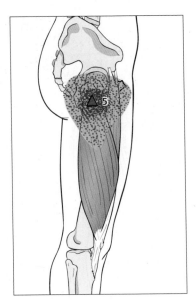

▲ Quadriceps Femoris Muscle, Knee Trigger Point

A non-myogenic trigger point is found at the insertion of the lateral collateral ligament of the knee joint. Here, the pain is found to radiate into the lateral femoral condyle.

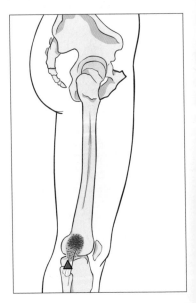

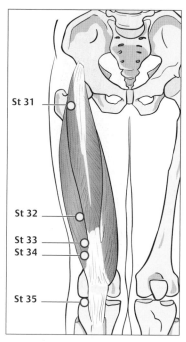

Important Acupuncture Points and Their Localizations

○ **St 31**

Location: With the hip flexed, in a depression lateral to the sartorius muscle at the intersection of the connecting line between the anterior superior iliac spine and lateral cranial pole of the patella, with the horizontal line through the lower border of the symphysis.

○ **St 32**

Location: 6 Cun above the upper lateral margin of the patella, on the line connecting the anterior superior iliac spine and lateral cranial pole of the patella.

○ **St 33**

Location: 3 Cun above the upper lateral margin of the patella, on the line connecting the anterior superior iliac spine and the lateral cranial pole of the patella.

○ **St 34**

Location: With the knee slightly bent, 2 Cun above the upper lateral margin of patella in a depression of the vastus lateralis muscle. The point lies on the line connecting the anterior superior iliac spine and lateral cranial pole of the patella.

○ **St 35**

Location: With the knee slightly bent, below the patella and lateral to the patellar tendon.

◎ Sp 10

Location: 2 Cun proximal to the medial cranial pole of the patella on the vastus medialis muscle in a depression that is often easy to palpate. Another way of localization: when placing the palm of the hand on the patella with the thumb slightly abducted, acupoint Sp 10 lies in front of the tip of the thumb.

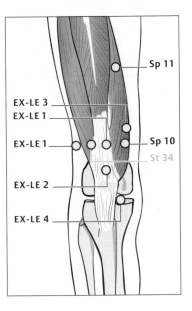

◎ Sp 11

Location: 6 Cun above acupoint Sp 10, lateral to the sartorius muscle in a depression between this muscle and the vastus medialis muscle.

◎ EX-LE 1 (Kuangu, Hip Bone)

Location: Two points left and right, 1.5 Cun next to acupoint St 34.

◎ EX-LE 2 (He Ding)

Location: In the middle of the upper margin of the patella.

◎ EX-LE 3 (Baichonwo, Warm Nest)

Location: 1 Cun above acupoint Sp 10 in the region of the vastus medialis muscle.

◎ EX-LE 4 (Nei Xi Yan)

Location: With the knee bent, in the depression medial to the patellar ligament in the region of the inner Knee Eye.

Description of the Muscle

Origin: Anterior surface of the sacrum.

Insertion: Tip of greater trochanter of femur.

Innervation: Sacral plexus (L5 to S2).

Action: Abducts the thigh and rotates it laterally.

Miscellaneous: In case of early division of the sciatic nerve, the common fibular nerve passes across the piriformis muscle and can be constricted here (piriformis syndrome).

Trigger Points of the Piriformis Muscle

Preliminary Remarks

The two trigger points of the piriformis muscle are often associated with chronic pain in the region of the loin, pelvis, and hip. They are activated by chronic disorders of the lumbosacral transition but only rarely as a reaction to acute strain. In cases where the muscle is shortened, entrapment of the sciatic nerve (especially of the peroneal portion) takes place in approximately 10 % of cases due to the aberrant course of the muscle; this should be considered in the differential diagnosis. Active associated trigger points of the inferior and superior gemellus muscles and of the obturator internus muscle appear regularly, as do those of the gluteus medius and gluteus maximus muscles.

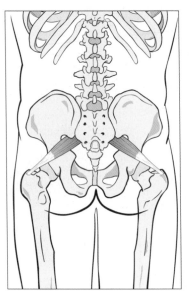

Examination of Trigger Points

Activation of trigger points is achieved by adducting the hip joint when flexed at 90° and simultaneously counter-rotating the remaining part of the spinal column. With the patient lying on his/her stomach, the piriformis muscle can be grasped by careful deep palpation between dorsal trochanter and sacrum.

Therapy of Trigger Points

Inactivation is possible by conventional acupuncture and dry-needling, and also by therapeutic local anesthesia. Passive stretching supported by postisometric relaxation decisively contributes to the success of treatment.

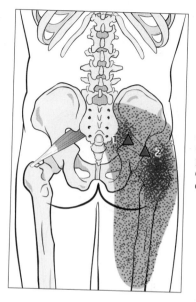

Trigger Points and Areas of Pain Projection

▲ Piriformis Muscle, Trigger Points 1 and 2

Trigger point 1 lies close to the insertion and has its main area of pain projection dorsal to the greater trochanter. By contrast, trigger point 2 lies close to the origin and has its projection area at the caudal pole of the sacroiliac joint. Both points share a common area of radiation over and beyond the buttocks into the dorsal thigh.

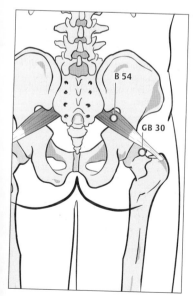

Important Acupuncture Points and Their Localizations

● B 54

Location: 3 Cun lateral to the sacral hiatus at the level of the 4th sacral foramen.

● GB 30

Location: Lateral side of the hip on the line connecting the greater trochanter and the sacral hiatus, between the outer and the middle third.

Description of the Muscle

Origin: Dorsal aspect of the ilium, thoracolumbar fascia, lateral edge of the sacrum and coccyx, sacrotuberal ligament.

Insertion: Gluteal tuberosity of the femur, iliotibial tract of the fascia lata, lateral intermuscular septum.

Innervation: inferior gluteal nerve (L4 to S1).

Action: Extends the thigh in the hip joint; upper fibers: abduction,
lower fibers: adduction, rotate the thigh laterally.

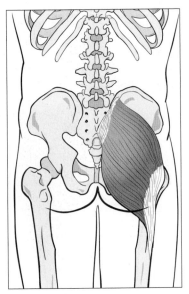

Trigger Points of the Gluteus Maximus Muscle

Preliminary Remarks

The muscle has three trigger points. Trigger points in this region often appear in combination with those of the gluteus minimus muscle and the sciaticocrural muscle. Trigger points of the deep dorsal extensor muscles are also found to be associated. Activation often results from acute events associated with increased strain of the gluteus maximus muscle. Such trigger points are therefore frequently found in athletes.

Examination of Trigger Points

The trigger points lie superficially and can easily be palpated. Local twitch responses are rarely observed. Especially in the case of trigger points 1 and 2, direct pressure sensibility of the sciatic nerve in the sense of Valleix's points should be differentiated.

Therapy of Trigger Points

Inactivation of trigger points is achieved without any problem by acupuncture, dry-needling, and therapeutic local anesthesia. Targeted stretching exercises using postisometric relaxation complete the treatment.

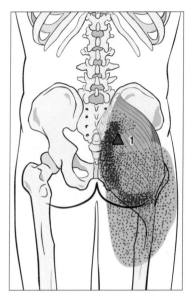

Trigger Points and Areas of Pain Projection

▲ **Gluteus Maximus Muscle, Trigger Point 1**

Trigger point 1 lies on the extension of a vertical line through the posterior iliac spine at the level of the proximal end of the gluteal fold; it has its main projection area along the medial and caudal margins of the muscle.

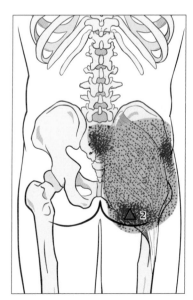

▲ **Gluteus Maximus Muscle, Trigger Point 2**

Trigger point 2 is found at the level of the caudal margin of the muscle approximately 4 to 5 cm above the gluteal crease. The projection areas are localized in this region, the entire gluteal region including the region over the caudal sacrum, and above the greater trochanter.

▲ Gluteus Maximus Muscle, Trigger Point 3

This point at the mediocaudal margin of the muscle has its main projection area in the direction of the coccyx.

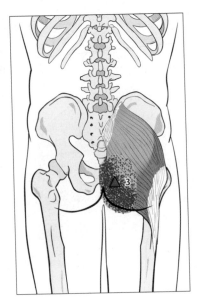

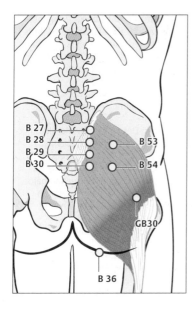

Important Acupuncture Points and Their Localizations

◉ B 27

Location: At the level of the first sacral foramen, 1.5 Cun lateral to the dorsal median line in a depression between the sacrum and upper region of the posterior superior iliac spine.

◉ B 28

Location: At the level of the 2nd sacral foramen, 1.5 Cun lateral to the dorsal median line.

◉ B 29

Location: At the level of the 3rd sacral foramen, 1.5 Cun lateral to the dorsal median line.

◉ B 30

Location: At the level of the 4th sacral foramen, 1.5 Cun lateral to the dorsal median line.

◉ B 36

Location: In the middle of the gluteal fold.

◉ B 53

Location: At the level of the 2nd sacral foramen, 1.5 Cun lateral to acupoint B 28.

◉ B 54

Location: At the level of the 4th sacral foramen, 3 Cun lateral to the sacral hiatus.

◉ GB 30

Location: On the lateral side of the hip joint, on the line connecting the greater trochanter and the sacral hiatus, between the outer and middle third.

Academy of Traditional Chinese Medicine (ed.): Essentials of Chinese Acupuncture. Foreign Languages Press, Beijing (VR China) 1980

Academy of Traditional Chinese Medicine (ed.): An Outline of Chinese Acupuncture. Foreign Languages Press, Beijing (VR China) 1975

Bachmann, G.: Die Akupunktur, eine Ordnungstherapie, Vol. 1. 3rd ed. Haug, Heidelberg 1980

Bahr, F. R.: Einführung in die wissenschaftliche Akupunktur. 6th ed. Vieweg, Braunschweig 1995

Bahr, F. R., Reis, A., Straube, E.-M., Strittmatter, B., Suwanda, S.: Skriptum für die Aufbaustufe aller Akupunkturverfahren. 4th ed. Eigenverlag, München, Deutsche Akademie für Akupunktur + Auriculomedizin e. V. 1993

Bergsmann, O., Bergsmann, R.: Projektionssyndrome. Facultas, Vienna 1988

Bergsmann, O., Bergsmann, R.: Projektionssymptome. 2nd ed. Facultas, Vienna 1990

Bischko, J.: Einführung in die Akupunktur, Vol. 1. 3rd ed. Haug, Heidelberg 1989

Bischko, J.: Akupunktur für mäßig Fortgeschrittene, Vol. 2. Haug, Heidelberg 1985

Bischko, J.: Weltkongress für wissenschaftliche Akupunktur, Kongreßband, Part 1. Vienna 1983

Bischko, J.: Sonderformen der Akupunktur. Broschüre 21.4.0 aus dem Handbuch der Akupunktur und Aurikulotherapie. Haug, Heidelberg 1981

Bucek, R.: Lehrbuch der Ohrakupunktur. Eine Synopsis der französischen, chinesischen und russischen Schulen. Haug, Heidelberg 1994

Chen Jing (ed.): Anatomical Atlas of Chinese Acupuncture Points. Shandong Science and Technology Press, Jinan (VR China) 1982

Chinese Traditional Medical College and Chinese Traditional Medical Research Institute of Shanghai (eds.): Anatomical Charts of the Acupuncture Points and 14 Meridians. People's Publishing House, Shanghai (VR China) 1976

DÄGfA: Akupunktur. Skripten Grundkurs I–III, 1995

Elias, J.: Lehrbuch- und Praxisbuch der Ohrakupunktur. Sommer, Tenningen 1990

Flows, Bob: Der wirkungsvolle Akupunkturpunkt. Verlag für Ganzheitliche Medizin Dr. E. Wühr, Kötzting 1993

Frick, H., Leonhardt, H., Starck, D.: Allgemeine Anatomie. Spezielle Anatomie I. Taschenbuch der gesamten Anatomie, Vol. 1. 3rd ed. Thieme, Stuttgart–New York 1987

Frick, H., Leonhardt, H., Starck, D.: Spezielle Anatomie II. Taschenlehrbuch der gesamten Anatomie, Vol. 2. 3rd ed. Thieme, Stuttgart 1987

Gerhard, I.: Die Ohrakupunktur. Technik und Einsatz in der Gynäkologie sowie Ergebnis bei Sterilitätsbehandlung. Erfahrungsheilkunde 39 (1990) 503–511

Gerhard, I., Müller, C.: Akupunktur in der Gynäkologie und Geburtshilfe. In: *Dittmer, Loch, Wiesenauer* (eds.): Naturheilverfahren in der Frauenheilkunde und Geburtshilfe. Hippokrates, Stuttgart 1994

Gerhard, I., Poostnek, F.: Möglichkeiten der Therapie durch Ohrakupunktur bei weiblicher Sterilität. Geburtsh. und Frauenheilk. 48 (1988) 154–171

Gleditsch, J. M.: Reflexzonen und Somatotopien als Schlüssel zu einer Gesamtschau des Menschen, 3rd ed. WBV Biologisch-Medizinische Verlagsgesellschaft, Schorndorf 1988

Gongwang, Liu (ed.): Acupoints & Meridians. Huaxia Publishing House Beijing 1996

Gray, H. et al.: Gray's Anatomy. 38th ed. Churchill Livingston, New York 1995

Hecker, U.: VISDAK, Visuell-didaktisches System – eine kombinierte Darstellung von Bild und Text auf dem Gebiet der Akupunktur und Naturheilkunde. Anmeldung Deutsches Patentamt München, 1997.

Hecker, U.: Ohr-, Schädel-, Mund-, Hand-Akupunktur, 2nd ed. Hippokrates, Stuttgart 1998

Hecker, U., Steveling, A.: Die Akupunkturpunkte. Hippokrates, Stuttgart 1997

Helms, J. M.: Acupuncture for the management of primary dysmenorrhea. Obstet. Gynecol. 69 (1987) 51–56

International Anatomical Nomenclature Committee: Nomina anatomica, 6th ed. Churchill Livingstone, Edinburgh 1989

Janda, V.: Manuelle Muskelfunktionsdiagnostik. 3rd ed. Ullstein-Mosby, Berlin 1994

Junghans, K.-H.: Akupunktur in der Geburtshilfe und Frauenheilkunde – ein Naturheilverfahren als "sanfte Alternative". Erfahrungsheilkunde 3 (1993) 114–123

Junghanns, K.-H.: Akupunktur in der Geburtshilfe und Gynäkologie – Bereicherung der Therapiemöglichkeiten. Therapiewoche, 43, 50 (1992) 2715–2720

Junghanns, K.-H.: Akupunktur in der Geburtshilfe – Behandlungsmöglichkeiten am Beispiel der Ohrakupunktur. Gyn.-Praktische Gynäkologie (1997) 434–450

Kampik, G.: Propädeutik der Akupunktur. Hippokrates, Stuttgart 1988

Kantoner militärsan. Einheit: Zhen Jiu Xue Wei Gua Tu Shuo Mind. Volksgesundheitsverlag der VR China

Kapandji, I. A.: Funktionelle Anatomie der Gelenke. 2nd ed. Enke, Stuttgart 1992

Kendall, Florence, Petersen, Kendall McCreary, Elisabeth: Muskeln, Funktion und Test. 2nd ed. G. Fischer, Stuttgart 1988

Kendall, F., Kendall, E.: Muscles Testing and Function. 3rd ed. Williams & Wilkins, Baltimore 1983

Kitzinger, E.: Der Akupunktur-Punkt. Maudrich, Vienna 1985

König, G., Wancura, I.: Einführung in die chinesische Ohrakupunktur. 9th ed. Haug, Heidelberg 1989

König, G.; Wancura, I.: Praxis und Theorie der Neuen chinesischen Akupunktur. Vol. 1 and 2. Vienna 1979/1983

König, G., Wancura, I.: Neue chinesische Akupunktur. Maudrich, Vienna 1985

Kropej, H.: Systematik der Ohrakupunktur. 7th ed. Haug, Heidelberg 1993

Kubiena, G., Meng, A.: Die neuen Extrapunkte in der chinesischen Akupunktur. Maudrich, Vienna 1994

Kubiena, G., Meng, A., Petricek, E., Petricek, U.: Handbuch der Akupunktur – der traditionell chinesische und der moderne Weg. Orac, Vienna 1991

Lange, G.: Akupunktur in der Ohrmuschel, Diagnostik und Therapie. WBV Biologisch-Medizinische Verlagsgesellschaft, Schorndorf 1985

Lang, J.: Klinische Anatomie des Kopfes. 1st ed. Springer, Berlin 1981

van Lanz, T., Wachsmuth, W.: Praktische Anatomie. Ein Lehrbuch und Hilfsbuch der anatomischen Grundlagen ärztlichen Handelns.
Vol. 1/1: Kopf. 1995
Vol. 1/2: Hals. 1995
Vol. 1/3: Arm. 3rd ed. 1996
Vol. 2/6: Bauch. 3rd ed. 1993
Springer, Berlin–Heidelberg–New York

Maciocia, G.: The foundations of Chinese medicine. Churchill Livingston, New York 1989

Marx, H.-G.: Medikamentfreie Entgiftung von Suchtkranken – Bericht über den Einsatz der Akupunktur. Suchtgefahren 30 (1984)

Nogier, P.-M.: Lehrbuch der Aurikulotherapie. Maisonneuve, Saint-Ruffine 1969

Petricek, E., Zeitler, H.: Neue systematische Ordnung der Neu-Punkte. Haug, Heidelberg 1976

Peuker, E. T., Filler, T. J.: Forensische Aspekte der Akupunktur – Eine Übersicht vor dem Hintergrund anatomischer Grundlagen. Ärztezeitschrift für Naturheilverfahren 38 (1997) 833–842

Peuker, E. T., Filler, T. J.: The need for practical courses in anatomy for acupuncturists. FACT 2 (1997) 194

Pöntinen, P. J., Gleditsch, J., Pothmann, R.: Triggerpunkte und Triggermechanismen. Hippokrates, Stuttgart 1997

Pothmann, R. (ed.): Akupunktur-Repetitorum. Hippokrates, Stuttgart 1992

Rampes, H., Peuker, E. T.: Adverse effects of acupuncture. In: *Ernst, E., White, A.* (ed.): Acupuncture: a scientific appraisal. Butterworth-Heinemann, Woburn MA 1999

Rauber, A., Kopsch, F.: Anatomie des Menschen, Vol. 2 and 4. Edited by H. Leonhardt, B. Tillmann, G. Töndury, K. Zilles. 20th ed. Thieme, Stuttgart–New York 1987

Roben, J.: Funktionelle Anatomie des Nervensystems. 4th ed. Schattauer, Stuttgart 1985

Rahen, J.: Funktionelle Anatomie des Menschen. 5th ed. Stuttgart 1987

Rohen, J.: Topographische Anatomie. 8th ed. Schattauer, Stuttgart 1987

Richter, K., Becke, H.: Akupunktur. Tradition, Theorie, Praxis. 2nd ed. Ullstein-Mosby, Berlin 1995

Rubach, A.: Principles of Ear Acupuncture. Thieme, Stuttgart 2001

Schmidt, H.: Konstitutionelle Akupunkturpunkte. Hippokrates, Stuttgart 1988

Schnorrenberger, C. C.: Die topographisch-anatomischen Grundlagen der chinesischen Akupunktur und Ohrakupunktur. 3rd ed. Hippokrates, Stuttgart 1983

Schnorrenberger, C. C.: Lehrbuch der chinesischen Medizin für westliche Ärzte. Die theoretischen Grundlagen der chinesischen Akupunktur und Arzneiverordnung. 3rd ed. Hippokrates, Stuttgart 1985

Sobotta-Becher: Atlas der Anatomie des Menschen, Vol. II. Edited by H. Ferner, J. Staubesand. 9th ed. Urban &

Schwarzenberg, Munich 1988

State Standard of the People's Republic of China (ed.): The Location of Acupoints. Foreign Languages Press, Beijing (VR China) 1990

Strauß, K. (ed.): Akupunktur in der Suchtmedizin. Hippokrates, Stuttgart 1997

Strittmatter, B.: Lokalisation der übergeordneten Punkte auf der Ohrmuschel. In: Der Akupunkturarzt/Aurikulotherapeut, edited by the Deutsche Akademie für Akupunktur und Aurikulomedizin e. V., Munich 1993

Stux, G., Stiller, N., Pomeranz, B.: Akupunktur – Lehrbuch und Atlas, 4th ed. Springer, Berlin–Heidelberg–New York 1993

Tillmann, B.: Farbatlas der Anatomie. Thieme, Stuttgart–New York 1997

Tittel, Kurt: Beschreibende und funktionelle Anatomie des Menschen. G. Fischer, Stuttgart 1990

Töndury, G.: Angewandte und topographische Anatomie. 5th ed. Thieme, Stuttgart–New York 1981

Travell, J. G., Simons, D. G.: Myofacial Pain and Dysfunction, Vol. 1 and 2. Williams & Wilkins, Baltimore 1992

Umlauf, R.: Zu den wissenschaftlichen Grundlagen der Aurikulotherapie. Dtsch. Z. Akupunktur 3 (1989) 59–65

Van Nghi, N.: Pathogenese und Pathologie der Energetik in der chinesischen Medizin, Vol. 1 and 2. Medizinisch-Literarische Verlagsgesellschaft mbH, Uelzen 1989/90

Wühr, E.: Quintessenz der chinesischen Akupunktur und Moxibustion. Lehrbuch der chinesischen Hochschule für Traditionelle Chinesische Medizin (German ed.). Verlag für Ganzheitliche Medizin Dr. E. Wühr, Kötzting 1988

■ Part 1: Body Acupuncture Points in Alphabetical Order

■ Part 2: Ear Acupuncture Points

Ear Points (Chinese Nomenclature) in Numerical Order

Ear Points (*Nogier* and *Bahr*) in Alphabetical Order

■ Part 3: Trigger Points in Alphabetical Order of the Muscles involved